Push your Career Publish your Thesis

Science should be accessible to everybody. Share the knowledge, the ideas, and the passion about your research. Give your part of the infinite amount of scientific research possibilities a finite frame.

Publish your examination paper, diploma thesis, bachelor thesis, master thesis, dissertation, or habilitation treatises in form of a book.

A finite frame by infinite science.

Infinite Science Publishing

An Imprint of
Infinite Science GmbH
MFC 1 | Technikzentrum Lübeck
BioMedTec Wissenschaftscampus
Maria-Goeppert-Straße 1
23562 Lübeck
book@infinite-science.de
www.infinite-science.de

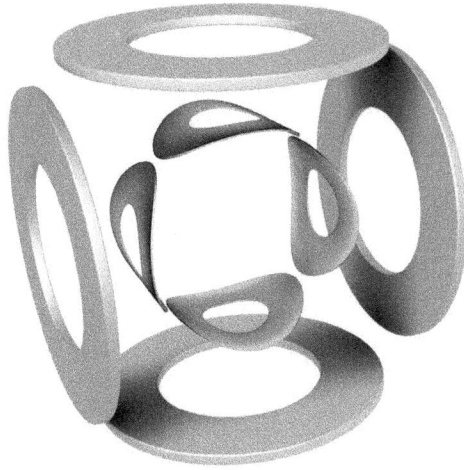

7th International Workshop on

Magnetic Particle Imaging
IWMPI 2017

March 23–24, 2017

Prague, Czech Republic

Book of Abstracts

L. Šefc, T. Knopp, and T. M. Buzug (Eds.)

Infinite Science
Publishing

© 2017 Infinite Science Publishing
  University Press and
  Academic Printig

Imprint of Infinite Science GmbH,
MFC 1 | BioMedTec Wissenschaftscampus
Maria-Goeppert-Straße 1
23562 Lübeck

Cover Design, Illustration: Uli Schmidts, metonym | Carsten Hinz, Infinite Science GmbH
Copy Editing: Infinite Science GmbH

Publisher: Infinite Science GmbH, Lübeck, www.infinite-science.de
Print: BoD, Norderstedt, Germany

ISBN Paperback: 978-3-945954-34-8

Bibliografische Information der Deutschen Nationalbibliothek:
Die Deutsche Nationalbibliothek verzeichnet diese Publikation in der Deutschen Nationalbibliografie; detaillierte bibliografische Daten sind im Internet über http://dnb.d-nb.de abrufbar.

Bibliographic information published by the Deutsche Nationalbibliothek
The Deutsche Nationalbibliothek lists this publication in the Deutsche Nationalbibliografie; detailed bibliographic data are available in the internet at http://dnb.d-nb.de.

Partner of IWMPI 2017

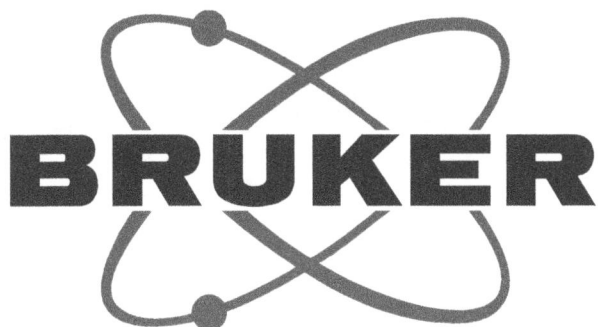

BRUKER

Exhibitors

nan⌀PET

pd PURE DEVICES
pure devices MAGNETIC RESONANCE IN SCIENCE

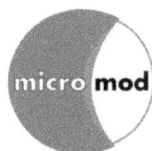

micro mod

OSYPKA
Technology for an active life

PACK LitzWire
for a better
power efficiency

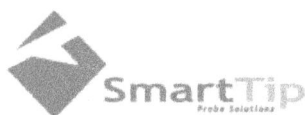

SmartTip
Probe Solutions

Infinite Science
Publishing

Support

Lacon

aselsan

Springer Vieweg

IOPscience

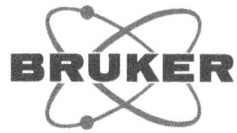

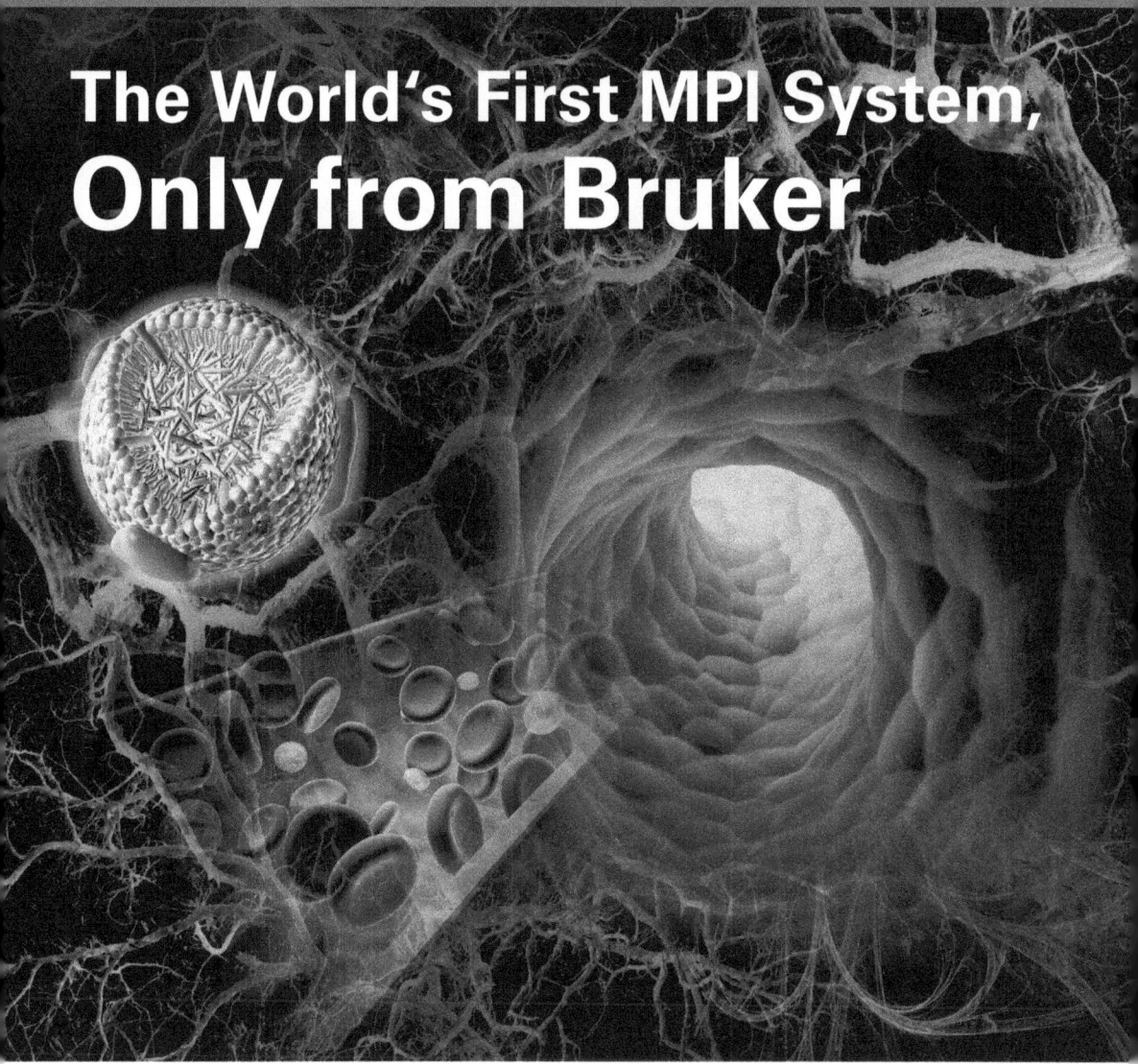

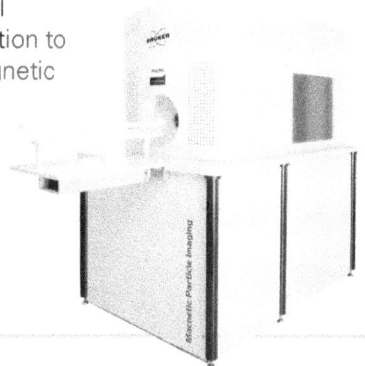

(12) INTERNATIONAL APPLICATION PUBLISHED UNDER THE PATENT COOPERATION TREATY (PCT)

(19) World Intellectual Property Organization
International Bureau

(43) International Publication Date
4 January 2007 (04.01.2007)

PCT

(10) International Publication Number
WO 2007/000350 A1

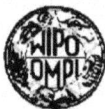

(51) International Patent Classification:
A61K 49/18 (2006.01)

(21) International Application Number:
PCT/EP2006/006319

(22) International Filing Date: 29 June 2006 (29.06.2006)

(25) Filing Language: English

(26) Publication Language: English

(30) Priority Data:
05014059.9   29 June 2005 (29.06.2005)   EP

(71) Applicant *(for all designated States except US)*: SCHER-ING AG [DE/DE]; Müllerstrasse 170-178, 13342 Berlin (DE).

(71) Applicant *(for all designated States except DE, US)*: KONINKLIJKE PHILIPS ELECTRONICS N.V. [NL/NL]; Groenewoudseweg 1, NL-5621 BA Eindhoven (NL).

(71) Applicant *(for DE only)*: PHILIPS INTELLECTUAL PROPERTY & STANDARDS GMBH [DE/DE]; Steindamm 94, 20099 Hamburg (DE).

(72) Inventors; and

(75) Inventors/Applicants *(for US only)*: BRIEL, Andreas [DE/DE]; Garnestrasse 10, 10245 Berlin (DE). GLE-ICH, Bernhard [DE/DE]; Rübenhofstrasse 41, 22335 Hamburg (DE). WEIZENECKER, Jürgen [DE/DE]; Reekamp 39, 22415 Hamburg (DE). ROHRER, Martin [DE/DE]; Victoriastrasse 13, 12203 Berlin (DE). WEIN-MANN, Hanns-Joachim [DE/DE]; Westhofener Weg

23, 14129 Berlin (DE). PIETSCH, Hubertus [DE/DE]; Ingwäonenweg 147, 13127 Berlin (DE). LAWACZECK, Rüdiger [DE/DE]; Beuschlaestrasse 8c, 13503 Berlin

(74)

(81)

(84) ... *kind of regional protection available)*: ARIPO (BW, GH, GM, KE, LS, MW, MZ, NA, SD, SL, SZ, TZ, UG, ZM, ZW), Eurasian (AM, AZ, BY, KG, KZ, MD, RU, TJ, TM), European (AT, BE, BG, CH, CY, CZ, DE, DK, EE, ES, FI, FR, GB, GR, HU, IE, IS, IT, LT, LU, LV, MC, NL, PL, PT, RO, SE, SI, SK, TR), OAPI (BF, BJ, CF, CG, CI, CM, GA, GN, GQ, GW, ML, MR, NE, SN, TD, TG).

Published:
— with international search report

For two-letter codes and other abbreviations, refer to the "Guidance Notes on Codes and Abbreviations" appearing at the beginning of each regular issue of the PCT Gazette.

(54) Title: COMPOSITIONS CONTAINING MAGNETIC IRON OXIDE PARTICLES, AND USE OF SAID COMPOSITIONS IN MAGNETIC PARTICLE IMAGING

(57) Abstract: The present invention relates to complexes which contain magnetic iron oxide particles in a pharmaceutically ac-cept... ...having a diameter of 20 nm to 1 μm with an overall particle diameter/core diameter ratio of less than 6, and ... (MPI). Particular preference is given to the use of these compositions in e... ...in the diagnosis of arteriosclerosis, infa...

WO 2007/000350 A1

mps

pd
pure devices

Magnetic Particle Spectrometer

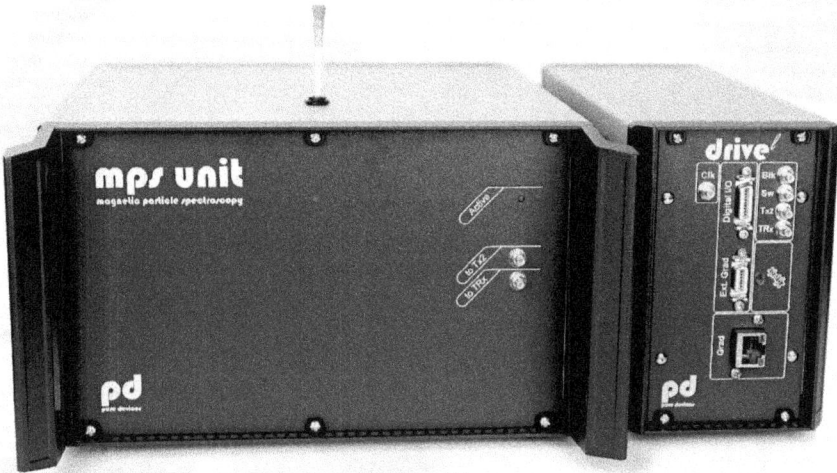

Characterization of

contrast agents
magnetic particles
MPI tracers
ferrofluides

Specifications

drive field: 0 - 30 mT
frequency: 20 kHz
bandwidth: 2.5 MHZ
test tubes: 6 mm

easy to set up

easy to operate

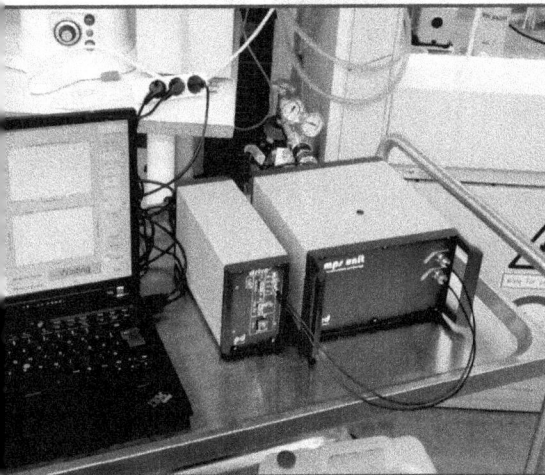

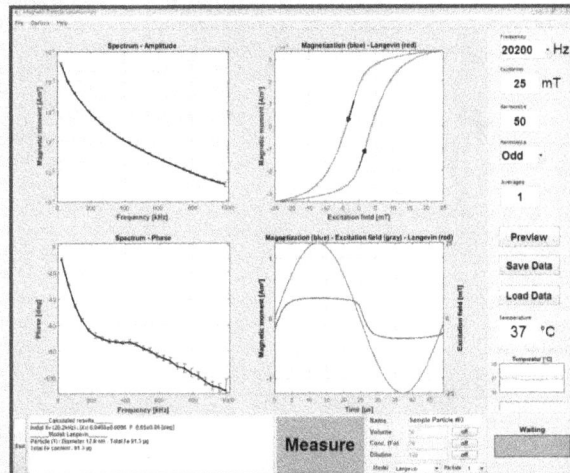

pd
pure devices

Pure Devices GmbH
Eisenbahnstr. 53
97084 Würzburg
GERMANY

www.pure-devices.com
info@pure-devices.com
Tel.: +49 (0) 931 71053590
Fax: +49 (0) 931 71053595

micromod **Partikeltechnologie GmbH**

For more than **20 years** micromod has been the reliable supplier of particle-based system components for *in vitro* diagnostics, high-throughput screening, magnetic bio-separation, cell labeling as well as a partner in R&D of novel components for diagnosis (MPI, MRI) and cancer therapy (hyperthermia). A modern quality management according to EN ISO 13485:2012/AC:2012 ensures a high quality standard in the development and production of **micro- and nanoparticles**.

perimag® - our new Magnetic Nanoparticles with Excellent Properties

➡ as contrast agent for Magnetic Particle Imaging (MPI)

➡ as contrast agent for Magnetic Resonance Imaging (MRI)

➡ for hyperthermia applications

➡ for homing and tracking of stem cells in regenerative medicine

Magnetic Particle Spectra:

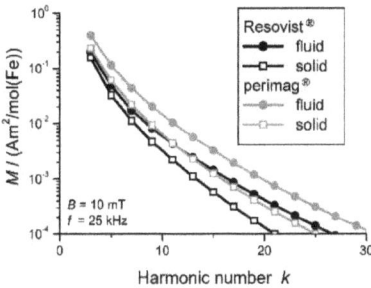

Magnetic Particle Spectra (MPS) of suspended and immobilized perimag® and Resovist® (D. Eberbeck *et al. IEEE Transactions on Magnetics* 2013, 49 (1) 269-274.)

Stem Cell Labeling with fluorescent perimag®:

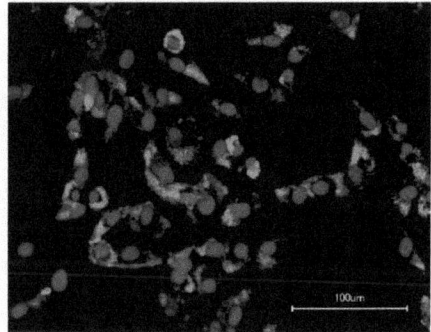

Labeling of hMSC with fluorescent perimag® (nucleus: blue; perimag® in cytoplasm: green) (M. Steinke et al. *Nanomedicine* 2016, 11 (15) 1957-1970.)

● The amplitude A3 of the 3rd harmonic in the MPS spectrum of perimag® is twice as high as that of Resovist®.

● Amino functionalized perimag® show high uptake in stem cells for MPI and MRI without use of transfection agents.

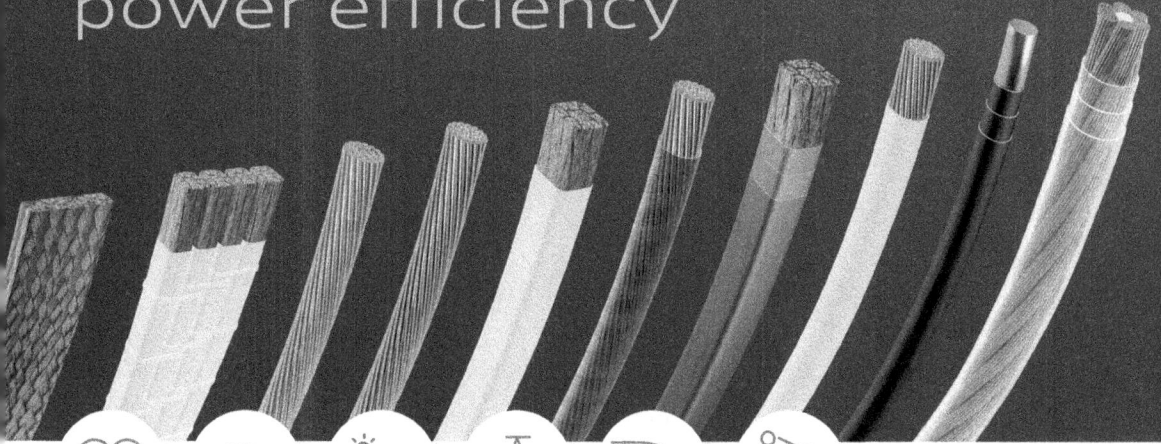

aselsan
research center

Vision Beyond Tomorrow

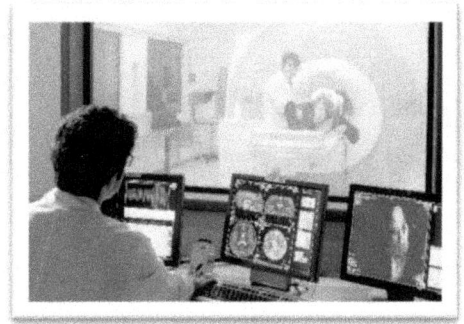

ASELSAN Research Center – as a part of the leading technology company in Turkey - conducts <u>applied research</u> activities for the future.

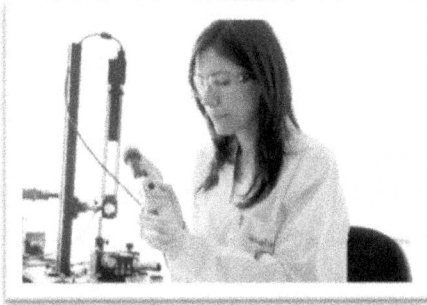

ASELSAN Research Center enhances the network between basic research activities in universities and product development activities in ASELSAN's engineering departments. In order to create an atmosphere that encourages creativity, it raises an innovative and cooperative research environment that gathers researchers, post-graduate students and scientists. Research studies are carried out by researchers and academicians specialized in their areas. Joint research programs are carried out with national/international universities, research centers and world's leading R&D companies to increase R&D know-how.

ASELSAN Research Center provides:

➢ An innovative and dynamic research environment,
➢ Opportunities for career development in academia,
➢ Development of novel technologies, concepts, patents and academic publications,
➢ Substantial funds for research projects,
➢ Active participation in international conferences and study groups,
➢ Effective collaborations with leading universities around the world.

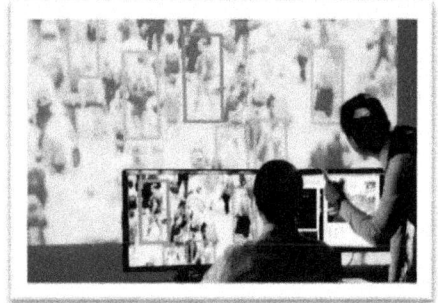

Technology Areas

+ Deep Learning
+ Data Analtytics
+ Medical Imaging
+ Compressive Sensing
+ Biotechnology
+ Signal and Image Processing

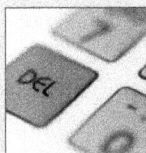

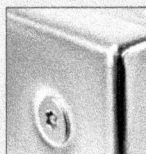

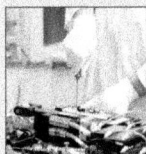

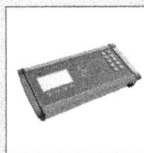

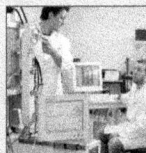

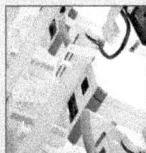

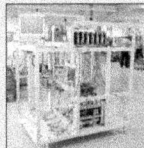

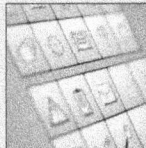

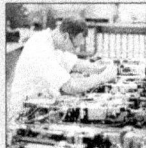

Scientific Committees

Workshop Chairs
Ludek Sefc · First Faculty of Medicine, Charles University · Czech Republic
Thorsten M. Buzug · University of Lübeck · Germany
Tobias Knopp · University Medical Center Hamburg (UKE) · Germany

Program Committee
G. Adam · UKE Hamburg · Germany
C. Alexiou · University of Erlangen · Germany
M. Asilturk · Akdeniz University · Turkey
J. Barkhausen · UKSH Lübeck · Germany
L. Bauer · Case Western Reserve University, Cleveland · USA
V. Behr · University of Würzburg · Germany
A. Bingolbali · Yildiz Technical University · Turkey
J. Bulte · John Hopkins University, Baltimore · USA
T. M. Buzug · University of Lübeck · Germany
S. M. Conolly · University of California, Berkeley · USA
N. Dogan · Gebze Technical University · Turkey
S. Dutz · TU Ilmenau · Germany
M. Ferguson · University of Washington · USA
D. Finas · EVKB Bielefeld · Germany
P. W. Goodwill · Magnetic Insight, Alameda · USA
J. Haueisen · Ilmenau University of Technology · Germany
M. Heidenreich · Bruker BioSpin, Ettlingen · Germany
U. Heinen · Pforzheim University of Applied Sciences · Germany
Y. Ishihara · Meiji University · Japan
P. Jakob · University of Würzburg · Germany
F. Kiesling · UKA Aachen · Germany
T. Knopp · UKE Hamburg and TU Hamburg-Harburg · Germany
K. Krishnan · University of Washington · USA
Liu W. · HUST, Wuhan · China
F. Ludwig · TU Braunschweig · Germany
M. Magnani · University of Urbino · Italy
K. Murase · Osaka University · Japan
J. Niehaus · CAN Hamburg · Germany
S. Odenbach · TU Dresden · Germany

Q. Pankhurst · University College London · GB

U. Pison · Charité Berlin · Germany

A. Samia · Case Western Reserve University, Cleveland · USA

E. U. Saritas · Bilkent University · Turkey

M. Schilling · Braunschweig University of Technology · Germany

J. Schnorr · Charité Berlin · Germany

L. Sefc · Charles University · Czech Republic

M. Taupitz · Charité Berlin · Germany

B. ten Haken · University of Twente · Netherlands

A. Tonyushkin · University of Massachusetts Bosten · USA

L. Trahms · PTB Berlin · Germany

J. Weaver · Dartmouth-Hitchcock Medical Center, Lebanon · USA

O. Weber · Philips Hamburg · Germany

A. Weis · University of Fribourg · Switzerland

J. Weizenecker · Karlsruhe University of Applied Sciences · Germany

F. Wiekhorst · PTB Berlin · Germany

B. Wollenberg · UKSH Lübeck · Germany

Preface and Acknowledgements

Dear Colleagues,

we are very pleased to host the 7th International Workshop on Magnetic Particle Imaging this year in Prague. We are proud to announce 60 contributions of participants from 10 countries in all fields of MPI namely Instrumentation, Application, Methodology, and Tracer Materials.

Since the first workshop in 2010, the International Workshop on MPI (IWMPI) has been the premier forum for researchers working in the MPI field. The workshop aims at covering the status and recent developments of both the instrumentation and the tracer material, as they are equally important in designing a well performing MPI system. The main topics presented at the workshop include hardware developments, image reconstruction and systems theory, nanoparticle physics and theory, nanoparticle synthesis, spectroscopy, patient safety, and medical/research applications of MPI.

We encourage you and your colleagues to contribute your research and results to the IWMPI, where you will have an opportunity to interact and collaborate with the greater MPI community, and to take steps in advancing the field of MPI. The workshop will provide a great opportunity to present your research results, as well as to learn more about the technical aspects and clinical potential of MPI.

In 2015, the International Journal on Magnetic Particle Imaging (IJMPI) has been launched as a future format for publishing high quality research articles on MPI (journal.iwmpi.org). The scope of the IJMPI ranges from imaging sequences and reconstruction over scanner instrumentation as well as particle synthesis and particle physics to pre-clinical and potential future clinical applications. Journal articles will be published online with open access under a Creative Commons License. In order to share ideas and experiences with a focused audience, we encourage submission of research papers to the new journal. IJMPI will publish research articles that can be submitted at any time.

As chairs of the workshop we would like to thank the members of the program committee for their exceptional service for the MPI community: G. Adam, University Medical Center Hamburg-Eppendorf (UKE); C. Alexiou, University Medical Center Erlangen; M. Asilturk, Akdeniz University, Antalya; J. Barkhausen, UKSH Lübeck; V. Behr, University of Würzburg; A. Bingolbali,

Yildiz Technical University, Istanbul; J. Bulte, John Hopkins University, Baltimore; T. M. Buzug, University of Lübeck; S. M. Conolly, University of California, Berkeley; N. Dogan, Gebze Institute of Technology, Kocaeli; S. Dutz, Technical University of Ilmenau; M. Ferguson, LodeSpin Labs, Seattle; D. Finas, Evangelisches Krankenhaus Bielefeld; P. W. Goodwill, University of California, Berkeley; M. Griswold, Case Western Reserve University, Cleveland; U. Häfeli, University of British Columbia, Vancouver; J. Haueisen, Technical University of Ilmenau; U. Heinen, Bruker BioSpin, Ettlingen; Y. Ishlhara, Meiji University, Tokyo; P. Jakob, University of Würzburg; T. Knopp, University Medical Center Hamburg- Eppendorf; K. Krishnan, University of Washington, Seattle; F. Ludwig, Technical University of Braunschweig; M. Magnani, University of Urbino; J. Niehaus, CAN Center for Applied Nanotechnology, Hamburg; S. Odenbach, Technical University of Dresden; U. Pison, Charité, Berlin; J. Rahmer, Philips GmbH Innovative Technologies, Hamburg; A. C. Samia, Case Western Reserve University, Cleveland; E. U. Saritas, Bilkent University, Bilkent/Ankara; M. Schilling, Technical University of Braunschweig; I. Schmale, Philips GmbH Innovative Technologies, Hamburg; J. Schnorr, Charité, Berlin; G. Schütz, Bayer HealthCare, Berlin; B. ten Haken, University of Twente, Enschede; L. Trahms, PTB, Berlin; J. B. Weaver, Dartmouth- Hitchcock Medical Center, Lebanon; J. Weizenecker, University of Applied Sciences, Karlsruhe; F. Wiekhorst, PTB, Berlin; B. Wollenberg, UKSH Lübeck.

Most importantly, we would like to thank our partners for their support and cooperation: Bruker BioSpin, nanoPET Pharma GmbH, Pure Devices GmbH, micromod Partikeltechnologie GmbH, SmartTip BV, PACK LitzWire, OSYPKA AG, ASELSAN A.Ş., Lacon Group, Oxford University Press, Springer-Vieweg, Infinite Science Publishing, DGBMT, Schwartau and would also like to extend our gratitude to the members of the local organization teams for their outstanding efforts and work.

We wish all of us an inspiring workshop and are already looking forward to IWMPI 2018 that will be held in Hamburg, Germany, March 22-24, 2018.

Ludek Sefc, Thorsten M. Buzug, and Tobias Knopp
Prague, March 2017

Program Overview

Thursday, March 23, 2017

08:45 – 17:30	**Registration**

09:15 – 11:30	**Tutorials**

09:15 – 10:15	**Tutorial I:** Instrumentation, Image Reconstruction in MPI
	V. Behr, P. Vogel
10:15 – 10:30	Coffee break
10:30 – 11:30	**Tutorial II:** Tracer Materials and Applications in MPI
	A. C. Samia

11:30 – 12:40	**Welcome** Luncheon and Coffee

12:40 – 12:50	**Opening Speech**
	L. Sefc, T. Knopp, T. Buzug

12:50 – 13:00	**Greetings**
	Prof. MUDr. Aleksi Šedo, DrSc.
	Dean of the First Faculty of Medicine,
	Charles University Prague

13:00 – 13:30	**Keynote 1:** Sentinel lymph node biopsy with a hand-held device using Differential Magnetometry *B. ten Haken; Magn. Det. & Imaging group, Fac. of Science & Technology, University of Twente, Enschede, The Netherlands* **Chair: T. Knopp**

13:30 – 14:30	**Session I: Instrumentation I** **Chair: L. Trahms**

13:30 – 13:45	Design analysis of an MPI human functional brain scanner *E. Mason*
13:45 – 14:00	Single-Sided Hybrid Selection Coils for Field-Free Line Magnetic Particle Imaging *A. Tonyushkin*
14:00 – 14:15	Towards a 2D MPI mechanical scanner based on atomic magnetometry *S. Colombo*
14:15 – 14:30	Novel Field Geometry featuring a Field Free Line for Magnetic Particle Imaging *M. Weber*
14:30 – 15:00	Coffee break

15:00 – 16:15	**Session II: Tracer Materials** **Chair: A. Samia**

15:00 – 15:15	A versatile MPI System Function Viewer *U. Heinen*
15:15 – 15:30	Effect of particle size and structure on harmonic intensity in blood-pooling multi-core magnetic nanoparticles for magnetic particle imaging *S. Ota*
15:30 – 15:45	Continuous synthesis of single core iron oxide nanoparticles for MPI tracer development *A. Baki*

15:45 – 16:00	Magnetic Particle Spectrometry of Microfabricated Magnetic Particles *Per A. Löthman*
16:00 – 16:15	Sensitivity Limits for in vivo ELISA Measurements of Molecular Biomarker Concentrations *John B. Weaver*
16:15 – 17:00	**Poster Session I** and Coffee
17:00 – 18:15	**Session III: Methodology I** **Chair: F. Ludwig**
17:00 – 17:15	SNR and Discretization Enhancement for System Matrix Determination by Decreasing the Gradient in Magnetic Particle Imaging *M. Graeser*
17:15 – 17:30	Applying Compressed Sensing on Hybrid System Matrices in Magnetic Particle Imaging *A. von Gladiß*
17:30 – 17:45	Model uncertainty in magnetic particle imaging: Motivating nonlinear problems by model-based sparse reconstruction *T. Kluth*
17:45 – 18:00	Improved image reconstruction in magnetic particle imaging using structural a priori information *C. Bathke*
18:00 – 18:15	Comparison of System-Matrix-Based and Projection-Based Reconstructions for Field Free Line Magnetic Particle Imaging *S. Ilbey*
19:00 – 22:30	Social Event
22:30 –	Fade-Out Drink at Lindner's Bar

Friday, March 24, 2017

09:00 – 10:15 **Session IV: Methodology II**
               Chair: U. Heinen

09:00 – 09:15 Influence of Orthogonal Receive Channels on the Spatial
               Resolution in Magnetic Particle Imaging

               P. Szwargulski

09:15 – 09:30 Improving the Spatial Resolution of Bidirectional Cartesian
               MPI Data using Fourier Techniques

               F. Werner

09:30 – 09:45 Selective Signal Suppression in MPI: Focusing on Areas of
               high Signal Intensity Range

               S. Herz

09:45 – 10:00 Artifact Analysis for Axially Elongated Lissajous Trajectories
               in Magnetic Particle Imaging

               C. Kaethner

10:00 – 10:15 Submillimeter Accurate Marker Localization within Low
               Gradient Magnetic Particle Imaging Tomograms

               F. Griese

10:15 – 11:00 **Poster Session II** and Coffee

11:00 – 11:30 **Keynote 2:** In vivo behaviour of SPION and how to modify
               their destiny
               M. Magnani, Università degli Studi "Carlo Bo", Urbino, Italy
               Chair: T. M. Buzug

11:30 – 12:45   **Session V: Methodology III**
                Chair: E. Saritas

11:30 – 11:45   Multifunctional SPIONs for Theranostics in Cancer

                S. Lyer

11:45 – 12:00   Magnetic nanoparticle temperature imaging with a 2D
                magnetic particle spectrometer scanner

                J. Zhong

12:00 – 12:15   Temperature-dependent MPS measurements

                S. Draack

12:15 – 12:30   Effects of Duty Cycle on Magnetostimulation Thresholds in
                MPI

                O. B. Demirel

12:30 – 12:45   Preparing system functions for quantitative MPI

                O. Kosch

12:45 – 13:00   Quo Vadis IJMPI

                T. Knopp

13:00 – 14:00   Lunch Break

14:00 – 15:00   **Session VI: Instrumentation II**
                Chair: J. Weaver

14:00 – 14:15   A Magneto Acoustic Spectrometer

                T. Friedrich

14:15 – 14:30   A summing confriguation based Low noise amplifier for
                MPI and MPS

                A. Malhotra

14:30 – 14:45   First measured result of the 3D Magnetic Particle
                Spectrometer

                X. Chen

14:45 – 15:00   Real-time 3D Dynamic Rotational Slice-Scanning Mode for
                Traveling Wave MPI

                P. Vogel

15:00 – 15:30   Coffee Break

15:30 – 17:00   **Session VII: Applications**
                Chair: L. Sefc

15:30 – 15:45   Towards the Integration of a Magnetic Particle Imaging
                Compatible Ultrasound Transducer

                T. C. Kranemann

15:45 – 16:00   Magnetic Particle Imaging of liver tumors in small animal
                models

                J. Dieckhoff

16:00 – 16:15   Detection of flow dynamic change in a 3D printed
                aneurysm model after treatment

                J. Sedlacik

16:15 – 16:30   MPI Flow Analysis Toolbox exploiting pulsed tracer
                information – an aneurysm phantom proof

                J. Franke

16:30 – 16:45   Relaxation-Based Viscosity Mapping in Different Viscous
                Enviroments

                M. Utkur

16:45 – 17:00   Determination of the Total Circulating Blood Volume using
                Magnetic Particle Spectroscopy

                F. Weigelt

17:00 – 17:30   Summary, Announcements for the CAPI Lab Tour and
                IWMPI 2018, Farewell

Saturday, March 25, 2017

	Lab Tour
	A lab tour through the Center for Advanced Preclinical
Group 1	Imaging (CAPI) including the new MPI installation is
09:30 – 10:30	organized by the local workshop chair Ludek Sefc, First
	Faculty of Medicine, Charles University Prague. Please do
Group 2	not forget to indicate your wish for participation on the lab
10:30 – 11:30	tour during registration. Places are restricted.

List of Posters

Applications

P01   Experimental and Simulation Studies on the Usefulness of Magnetic Particle Imaging for Monitoring the Effect of Magnetic Targeting
K. Murase, Osaka University

P02   Magnetic Nanoparticle-Gel Materials for Development of MPI and MRI Phantoms
S. Dutz, TU Ilmenau

P03   Magnetic Particle Imaging for clinical cardiovascular imaging
J. Haegele, University Medical Center SH, Luebeck

P04   Seamless Integration of MPI into a Small Animal Imaging Unit at the Center for Advanced Preclinical Imaging Prague
L. Sefc, Charles University Prague

Instrumentation

P05   Simulation Study of Novel Selection-Focus Field Coils for Field-Free Line Magnetic Particle Imaging
A. Tonyushkin, University of Massachusetts Boston

P06   Experimental Validation of the Selection Field of a Rabbit Sized FFL Scanner
A. Bakenecker, University of Luebeck

P07   Spectral Measurements Inside a Rabbit Sized FFL-MPI Device Using a Gradiometric Receive Coil
J. Stelzner, University of Luebeck

P08   Differential magnetometry to detect sentinel lymph nodes in laparoscopic procedures
M. van de Loosdrecht, University of Twente

Tracer Materials

P18   MPS and MRI efficacy of magnetosomes from wild-type and mutant
        bacterial strains
        D. Heinke, nanoPET Pharma GmbH

P19   Synthesis and Characterisation of Superparamagnetic Polylactic acid
        based Polymers
        K. Lüdtke-Buzug, University of Luebeck

P20   Resolution study on new MPI tracer material
        C. Debbeler, University of Luebeck

P21   Linearized spectra of Preclinical MPI scanner for tracer characterization
        O. Kosch, PTB, Germany

P22   Magnetic Particle Spectrometry of Fe3O4 nanoclustered particles
        L. Abelmann, KIST Europe

P23   Continuous synthesis of single core iron oxide nanoparticles for MPI
        tracer development
        A. Baki; Fraunhofer ICT-IMM

Tutorials

The workshop will start with two tutorials to provide a thorough introduction to Instrumentation and Image Reconstruction in MPI as well as Tracer Materials and Applications in MPI to those new in the field of Magnetic Particle Imaging.

Tutorial I: Instrumentation and Image Reconstruction in MPI

Thursday, March 23, 2017, 09:15 – 10:15

PD Dr. Volker Christian Behr
and Dr. Patrick Vogel

University of Würzburg, Germany

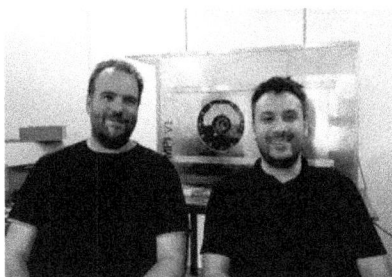

Tutorial II: Tracer Materials and Applications in MPI

Thursday, March 23, 2017, 10:30 - 11:30

Anna Cristina Samia

Case Western Reserve University, Cleveland, USA

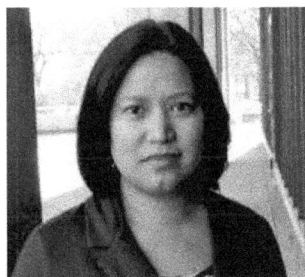

Tutorial I: Instrumentation and Image Reconstruction in MPI

Thursday, March 23, 2017, 09:15 – 10:15

Volker Christian Behr and Patrick Vogel
University of Würzburg, Germany

What do you need for building and operating your own MPI scanner?
In this tutorial we will take you on a journey starting from the basic concept of a Magnetic Particle Imaging scanner to the reconstructed images.

Several scanner designs have been presented since the first introduction of MPI in 2005. However, all systems are relying on the same physical principle, the non-linear magnetization response of magnetic materials to alternating magnetic fields.

Different scanner topologies based on field-free points or field-free lines will be introduced and we will discuss how they generate and acquire signal. Individual components of the signal chain of an MPI scanner (e.g. field and receive coils, filters, etc.) will be illustrated leading the participants as an example to a fully operational TWMPI system. A special focus will be typical issues arising when implementing such a device and how they are overcome.

In the second part an overview of the processing of the data, especially of the reconstruction will be given.

We will discuss different reconstruction strategies with respect to correction steps necessary to prepare the acquired signal, gridding, deconvolution or reconstruction using system matrices. Advantages and disadvantages of both of the latter concepts will be compared. Furthermore, steps to accelerate the reconstruction processes will be shown since the high temporal resolution of MPI itself promises access to real-time imaging.

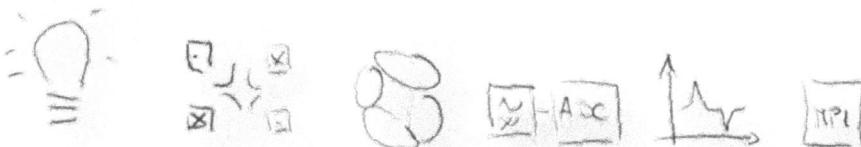

Tutorial II: Tracer Materials and Applications in MPI

Thursday, March 23, 2017, 10:30 - 11:30

Anna Cristina Samia

Case Western Reserve University, Cleveland, USA

In MPI, the development of tailored magnetic nanoparticle tracers is paramount to achieving high sensitivity and good spatial resolution. This tutorial will provide a general overview of the progress in MPI tracer development over the past decade, and will also focus on emerging directions and new opportunities for iron oxide-based tracer design and applications.

The presentation will cover magnetic nanoparticle relaxation in MPI and discuss key aspects to consider in tailoring tracers for MPI applications. Emphasis will be given on how structural changes (size, composition, shape, surface chemistry) and inter-particle interactions affect the MPI signal generation process. Moreover, the presentation will discuss emerging research directions in color-MPI (cMPI) and MPI- guided hyperthermia (hMPI).

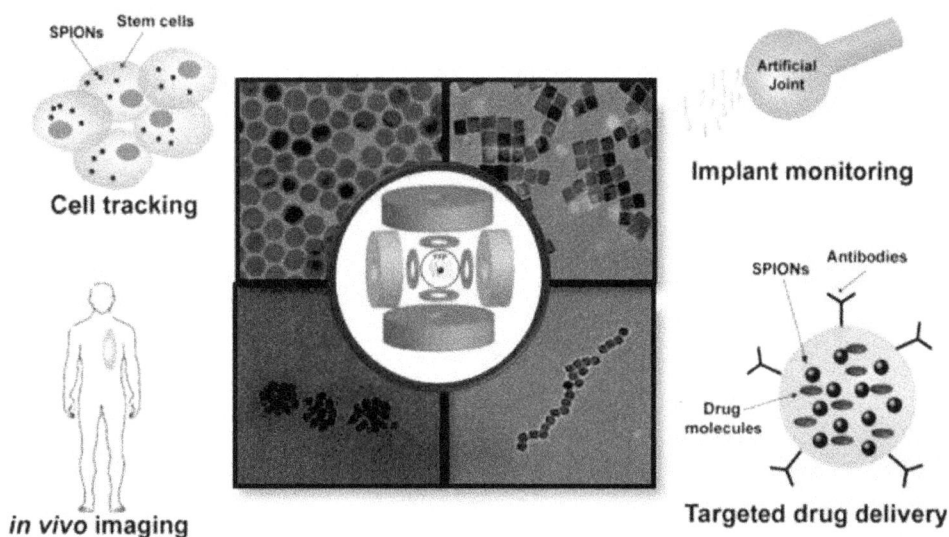

Contents

Poster – Applications

Poster – Instrumentation

Poster – Methodology

Poster – Tracer Materials

Methodology I

Methodology II

Applications

Keynote 1

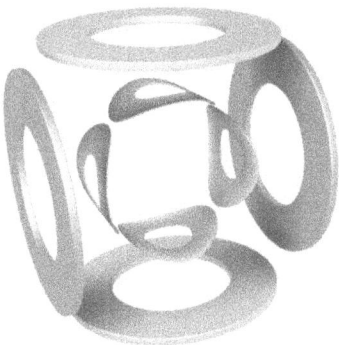

Sentinel Lymph Node Biopsy with a Hand-Held Device using Differential Magnetometry

Bennie ten Haken

Magnetic Detection & Imaging Group
University of Twente, Enschede, The Netherlands

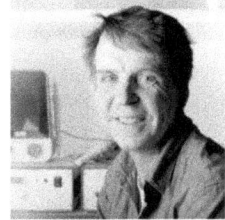

Sentinel lymph node biopsy is a vital procedure in the staging of breast cancer. By replacing the morbidity-plagued axillary node clearance with removing only those nodes most likely to contain metastases, it has greatly improved the quality of life of many breast cancer patients. However, due to the use of ionizing radiation emitted by the technetium-based tracer material, the current sentinel lymph node biopsy has serious drawbacks. Magnetic alternatives have been tested in recent years, but all have their own drawbacks, mostly related to interference from metallic instruments and the natural magnetism of the human body. In this presentation, we demonstrate an MPI-based approach that utilizes the unique nonlinear magnetic properties of superparamagnetic iron oxide nanoparticles. Contrary to many other nonlinear magnetic approaches the required field amplitudes are limited to 5 mT, which enables handheld operation without additional cooling. We show that excellent mass sensitivity can be obtained without the need for external re-balancing of the probe to negate any influences from the magnetism of the human body. Additionally, we show how this approach can be used to suppress artefacts resulting from the presence of metallic instruments, which are a significant deal-breaker when using a conventional magnetometer, MPI or MRI. We present our new research on two pathologies where the radio-isotope approach appeared to be non-successful. Head and neck squamous cell carcinoma (HNSCC) is the seventh most common cancer type worldwide, accounting for approximately 4% of all malignant tumors. The complex anatomy of the head and neck region poses technical challenges, and complicates the introduction of this technique for head and neck cancer patients, especially in floor of mouth carcinomas. The second case involves laparoscopic surgery, where the size limitation of the detector (~12 mm) imposes an important hurdle for magnetic sensing with a handheld instrument.

Session I

Instrumentation I

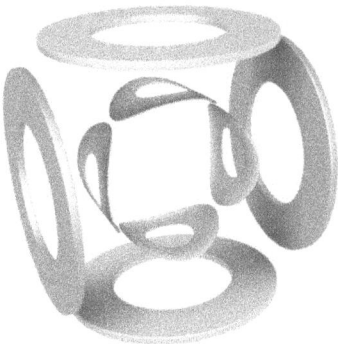

Design analysis of an MPI human functional brain scanner

E. Mason[* a,c)], C. Z. Cooley[a)], S. F. Cauley[a)], M. A. Griswold[d)],
S. M. Conolly[e)], L. L. Wald[a,b)]

a) MGH-HST A.A. Martinos Center for Biomedical Imaging, Dept. of Radiology,
Massachusetts General Hospital, Charlestown, MA, USA
b) Harvard Medical School, Boston, MA, USA
c) Harvard-MIT Health Sciences and Technology, Cambridge, MA, USA
d) Case Western Reserve University, OH, USA
e) University of California, Berkeley, CA, USA
[*]Corresponding author, email: emason1@mgh.harvard.edu

MPI's high sensitivity makes it a promising modality for imaging brain function. Functional contrast is proposed based on blood SPION concentration changes due to Cerebral Blood Volume (CBV) increases during activation, a mechanism utilized in fMRI studies. MPI offers the potential for a direct and more sensitive measure of SPION concentration, and thus CBV, than fMRI. As such, fMPI could surpass fMRI in sensitivity, enhancing the scientific and clinical value of functional imaging.

As human-sized MPI systems have not been attempted, we assess the technical challenges of scaling MPI from rodent to human brain. We use a full-system MPI simulator to test arbitrary hardware designs and encoding practices, and we examine tradeoffs imposed by constraints that arise when scaling to human size as well as safety constraints (PNS and central nervous system stimulation) not considered in animal scanners, thereby estimating spatial resolutions and sensitivities achievable with current technology.

Using a projection FFL MPI system, we examine coil hardware options and their implications for sensitivity and spatial resolution. We estimate that an fMPI brain scanner is feasible, although with reduced sensitivity (20x) and spatial resolution (5x) compared to existing rodent systems. Nonetheless, it retains sufficient sensitivity and spatial resolution to make it an attractive future instrument for studying the human brain; additional technical innovations can result in further improvements.

Single-Sided Hybrid Selection Coils for Field-Free Line Magnetic Particle Imaging

A. Tonyushkin

Physics Department, University of Massachusetts Boston, Boston, MA, USA
email: alexey.tonyushkin@umb.edu

Single-sided Magnetic Particle Imaging (MPI) is a promising new development that can help translating MPI technology into clinical practice. Unlike currently available closed geometry MPI scanners single-sided device does not have a hardware around the object thus providing unlimited access to the field of view from one of the sides. The major progress includes a demonstration of 2D imaging on a single-sided device that utilizes a field-free point coplanar coil topology. Previously, we proposed a design of a field-free line selection field generator for a single-sided geometry. Here, we extend our single-sided design to incorporate a much more efficient scheme that utilizes permanent magnets.

Towards a 2D MPI mechanical scanner based on atomic magnetometry

S. Colombo[* a)], V. Lebedev[a)], A. Tonyushkin[b)], Z. D. Grujic[a)],
V. Dolgovskiy[a)], A. Weis[a)]

a) Physics Department, University of Fribourg, Fribourg, Switzerland
b) Physics Department, University of Massachusetts Boston, Boston, MA, USA
[*]Corresponding author, email: simone.colombo@unifr.ch

We report on our progress in the development of an atomic magnetometer (AM) based low-frequency X-space MPI scanner, expected to be free from SAR and PNS constraints. We address major challenges in coil and sensor design due to specific AM properties. Compared to our previous work we have changed the AM's mode of operation towards its implementation for detecting weak SPIO response fields in the presence of nearby-located strong drive/selection fields. We demonstrate that a pump-probe AM scheme in a buffer gas filled alkali vapour cell can tolerate mT/m gradients while maintaining a sensitivity in the one-digit $pT/Hz^{1/2}$ range over a bandwidth from DC to several kHz. We give a detailed description of the drive/selection coils' geometry and their hardware implementations that will provide both field-free-line (FFL) and field-free-point (FFP) modes of operation, compatible with a best performance AM operation. We estimate the achievable field of view and spatial resolution of the scanner as well as its sensitivity, assuming mechanical scanning of a Resovist sample through the field-free point/line.

Novel Field Geometry featuring a Field Free Line for Magnetic Particle Imaging

M. Weber[*], T. M. Buzug

Institute of Medical Engineering, Universität zu Lübeck, Lübeck, Germany
[*]Corresponding author, email: {weber,buzug}@imt.uni-luebeck.de

The complexity of the imaging device in Magnetic Particle Imaging (MPI) using a field free line (FFL) is the biggest challenge in realizing such devices. This is especially the case for systems featuring large bores, high gradients or high temporal resolution. In this work, we suggest a novel Halbach cylinder based field generator that is able to generate an FFL with a gradient of 5 T/m. By rotating the Halbach array, FFL projections can be acquired. Furthermore, just one static drive field coil is needed for two-dimensional imaging. The presented concept could combine high gradient strength and high temporal resolution with minimum space requirements for FFL-MPI imaging in the future.

Session II

Tracer Materials

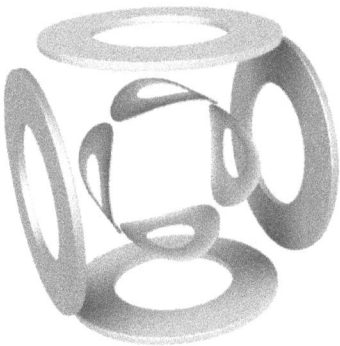

A versatile MPI System Function Viewer

U. Heinen[* a], A. Weber[b], J. Franke[b], H. Lehr[b], O. Kosch[c]

a) University of Applied Sciences Pforzheim, Pforzheim, Germany
b) Bruker Biospin MRI GmbH, Ettlingen, Germany
c) Physikalisch-Technische Bundesanstalt, Berlin, Germany
*Corresponding author, email: ulrich.heinen@hs-pforzheim.de

Magnetic Particle Imaging (MPI) is a versatile new imaging technique for mapping the spatial distribution of magnetic nanoparticle (MNP) based tracers in vivo and in real time with high sensitivity. Reconstruction of 3D-encoded MPI data with high temporal resolution so far relies on the so-called system matrix approach. Here, the image is obtained by solving a linear system of equations involving pre-measured data from a point sample moved over the later reconstruction grid. A study of these pre-measured data, or system matrices, is a useful way of gaining insight into the MNP properties. Unfortunately, the size of the datasets, which easily reaches dozens of gigabytes, presents an obstacle for a visual inspection and analysis. Here we present a tool for convenient inspection of MPI system functions with versatile navigation and visualization features.

Effect of particle size and structure on harmonic intensity in blood-pooling multi-core magnetic nanoparticles for magnetic particle imaging

S. Ota[* a)], R. Takeda[b)], T. Yamada[b)], I. Kato[c)], S. Nohara[c)],
Y. Takemura[b)]

a) Department of Electrical and Electronic Engineering, Shizuoka University, Hamamatsu, Japan
b) Department of Electrical and Computer Engineering, Yokohama National University, Yokohama, Japan
c) The Nagoya Research Laboratory, Meito Sangyo Co., Ltd., Kiyosu, Japan
*Corresponding water, email: ota.s@shizuoka.ac.jp

Magnetic particle imaging has been developed by the optimization of the tracer materials, excitation systems, and system functions for image reconstruction. Here, we prepared and studied magnetic nanoparticles with different core diameters, coated by carboxymethyl-diethylaminoethyl dextran as a blood-pooling agent. For comparison, measurements were also performed using Resovist®, a widely used tracer agent. Transmission electron microscopy analysis of the prepared samples of nanoparticles revealed monodisperse single-core, chainlike aggregation, and multi-core structures. For optimizing the core size and structure of magnetic nanoparticles for use as imaging tracers, we evaluated the magnetization response to an applied field and harmonic intensity by measuring direct and alternating current hysteresis loops. To evaluate the dependence of the harmonic intensity on the core size and particle structures, large-magnetization particles were assembled using magnetic separation. The harmonic intensity depended not only on the core size but also on the particle structure. Diameters and distributions of single- and multi-core particles are important parameters. Solid and liquid samples of particles were studied for characterization of imaging of solid objects (such as tumors and organs) and liquids (such as blood).

Continuous synthesis of single core iron oxide nanoparticles for MPI tracer development

A. Baki [a], N. Löwa [b], R. Thiermann [a], C. Bantz [a], M. Maskos [a], F. Wiekhorst [b], R. Bleul[*] [a]

a) Fraunhofer ICT-IMM, Mainz, Germany
b) Physikalisch-Technische Bundesanstalt, Berlin, Germany
*Corresponding author, email: regina.bleul@imm.fraunhofer.de

The development of suitable tracers with optimized characteristics is a crucial factor to bring the powerful and high-innovative technology of Magnetic Particle Imaging further towards clinics. Successful engineering of new magnetic particles for this imaging method requires a deeper understanding of structure-performance relationships. Even though many international research groups work in the field of tracer development for the MPI technology, until now no economic and reproducible synthesis method was found to produce high-performance tracer materials with optimal characteristics. In the present work recent achievements in the continuous synthesis of single-core iron oxide nanoparticles with tunable characteristics employing a micromixer set-up are reported.

Magnetic Particle Spectrometry of Microfabricated Magnetic Particles

P. A. Löthman [a], T. Janson [a], Y. Klein [a], A.-R. Blaudszun [a], M. Ledwig [b], L. Abelmann [*a]

a) Korea Institute of Science and Technology Europe, Saarbrücken, Germany
b) Pure Devices, Würzburg, Germany
*Corresponding author, email: L.Abelmann@kist-europe.de

We report on the fabrication of dispersions of Au/Ni81Fe19/Au magnetic discs with two and three micrometer diameter and thickness in the order of hundred nanometers. The magnetization reversal of the discs was analyzed on a time-scale of an hour and a few milliseconds, to assess their suitability for magnetic particle imaging. We conclude that compared to FeraSpin particles, these microfabricated particles saturate in fields as low as 12 mT, the shape of the hysteresis loop is relatively independent on the field sweep rate, and the difference in phase between higher harmonics is constant up to the 20th harmonic. These radically different magnetic properties suggest that that microfabricated particles might have advantages for applications such as magnetic particle imaging.

Sensitivity Limits for in vivo ELISA Measurements of Molecular Biomarker Concentrations

J. B. Weaver[* a,b,c], Y. Shi[b], D. B. Ness[a], H. Khurshid[a],
A. C. S. Samia[d]

a) Department of Radiology, Dartmouth-Hitchcock Medical Center and the Geisel School of Medicine, Dartmouth College
b) Department of Physics, Dartmouth College
c) Thayer School of Engineering, Dartmouth College
d) Department of Chemistry, Case Western Reserve University
*Corresponding author, email: john.b.weaver@dartmouth.edu

The extremely high sensitivity that has been suggested for magnetic particle imaging has its roots in the unique signal produced by the nanoparticles at the frequencies of the harmonics of the drive field. That sensitivity should be translatable to other methods that utilize magnetic nanoparticle probes, specifically towards magnetic nanoparticle spectroscopy that is used to measure molecular biomarker concentrations for an "in vivo ELISA" assay approach. In this paper, we translate the predicted sensitivity of magnetic particle imaging into a projected sensitivity limit for a magnetic nanoparticle spectroscopy based in vivo ELISA approach. The simplifying assumptions adopted are: 1) the limiting noise in the detection system is equivalent to the minimum detectable mass of nanoparticles; 2) the nanoparticle's signal arising from Brownian relaxation is completely eliminated by the molecular binding event, which can be accomplished by binding the nanoparticle to something so massive that it can no longer physically rotate. Given these assumptions, the equation for the minimum concentration of molecular biomarker we should be able to detect is obtained and the in vivo sensitivity is estimated to be in the attomolar to zeptomolar range.

Poster Session
Applications

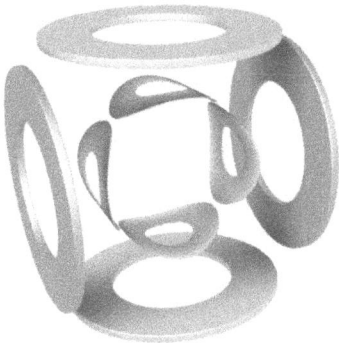

Experimental and Simulation Studies on the Usefulness of Magnetic Particle Imaging for Monitoring the Effect of Magnetic Targeting

N. Banura, K. Murase[*]

Department of Medical Physics and Engineering, Osaka University Graduate School of Medicine, Osaka, Japan
*Corresponding author, email: murase@sahs.med.osaka-u.ac.jp

Methods for magnetic targeting have been developed for localizing drug carriers in targeted organs or tissues by applying an external magnetic gradient field for improving the therapeutic effect of drugs and minimizing the unwanted side effects. In this study, we applied magnetic particle imaging (MPI) to monitoring the effect of magnetic targeting and investigated its usefulness. First, we performed phantom experiments for aerosol-based magnetic targeting using a simple flow model, in which the dependencies of the targeting efficiency on physical parameters such as flow rate and magnetic field were investigated using MPI. Second, we performed simulation studies based on computational fluid dynamics (CFD). Finally, we evaluated the usefulness of MPI for monitoring the effect of magnetic targeting by comparing the experimental and simulation results.

Magnetic Nanoparticle-Gel Materials for Development of MPI and MRI Phantoms

A. Mattern [a], R. Sandig [a], A. Joos [b], N. Löwa [b], O. Kosch [b], A. Weidner [a], F. Wiekhorst [b], S. Dutz[*] [a]

a) Institute of Biomedical Engineering and Informatics, Technische Universität Ilmenau, Ilmenau, Germany
b) Physikalisch-Technische Bundesanstalt, Berlin, Germany
*Corresponding author, email: silvio.dutz@tu-ilmenau.de

To evaluate performance of commercial as well as various custom-made scanners in several laboratories, dedicated phantoms with defined magnetic nanoparticle (MNP) distributions are required. Pre-requirement for the development of such phantoms is the establishment of suitable MNP-matrix combinations. In this study, two different gel types were used as matrix materials, which show similar imaging behavior in MRI and MPI compared to body tissue: water based biopolymers and synthetic polymers. Aqueous suspensions of MNP coated with different types of functionalized dextranes were used for embedding particles into the biopolymers, and organic fluids with oleic acid coated MNP for synthetic polymers, respectively. The obtained MNP-matrix combinations were tested for their mechanical stability by means of mechanical load tests. The homogeneity of MNP distribution and immobilization within the matrix was determined by optical investigation of the samples with a microscope and by investigation of the magnetic particle properties measured by vibrating sample magnetometry. In summary, we found suitable combinations of coated magnetic nanoparticles and matrix materials for the buildup of MPI phantoms, which guarantee a fixation of the MNP within the matrix without agglomeration of the particles.

Magnetic Particle Imaging for clinical cardiovascular imaging

F. Wegner, S. Vaalma, N. Panagiotopoulos, F. M. Vogt,
J. Barkhausen, J. Haegele[*]

University Medical Center Schleswig-Holstein, Lübeck, Germany
*Corresponding author, email: Julian.Haegele@uksh.de

Recent preclinical data proof, that cardiovascular imaging is a promising application for Magnetic Particle Imaging (MPI). The proof of concept for cardiovascular imaging in larger animals and humans is missing. For that, the field of view has to be enlarged without diminishing the spatial and temporal resolution. While this is technically possible, safety aspects like peripheral nerve stimulation and patient heating have to be considered. To be an alternative or a reasonable addition to existing methods like CT and MRI, MPI has to meet the requirements for the application scenarios in clinical imaging, which are defined in guidelines by the professional societies. In this work, the requirements for clinical cardiac CT and MRI are reviewed based on the consensus statements and guidelines by the Society of Cardiac Computed Tomography (SCCT) and the Society for Cardiovascular Magnetic Resonance. It is discussed how MPI can meet these requirements, where MPI can add to these methods and where it is sensible to deviate from the requirements due to the unique features of MPI.

Seamless Integration of MPI into a Small Animal Imaging Unit at the Center for Advanced Preclinical Imaging Prague

L. Sefc[*], P. Francova, V. Kolarova, V. Sykora

Center for Advanced Preclinical Imaging (CAPI), First Faculty of Medicine, Charles University, Prague, Czech Republic
*Corresponding author, email: sefc@cesnet.cz

Center for Advanced Preclinical Imaging (CAPI) in Prague was opened in February, 2016 as the first multimodal imaging center in the Czech Republic and Eastern Europe. The following modalities are employed: CT, MRI, PET, SPECT, Cherenkov radiation, fluorescence, luminescence, and MPI. Ultrasound and photoacoustics will be installed within few months. The laboratories have a GMO approval and currently are in a process of GLP certification. CAPI is a part of CzechBioImaging, a member of EuroBioImaging. All imaging devices are hardware and software compatible that allows a true multimodal imaging performed on a single anesthetized animal. CAPI serves as a core facility but it also performs its own research. Multiple cooperation exists including multimodal MPI/PET/OI and MPI/PA tracer development. The lab tour will be offered after IWMPI meeting.

Poster Session

Instrumentation

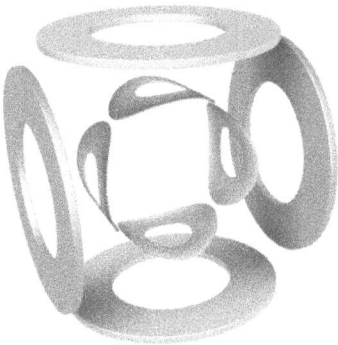

Simulation Study of Novel Selection-Focus Field Coils for Field-Free Line Magnetic Particle Imaging

A. Tonyushkin

Physics Department, University of Massachusetts Boston, Boston, MA, USA
email: alexey.tonyushkin@umb.edu

Magnetic particle imaging (MPI) shows great promise for various medical imaging applications. A major challenge for future applications are contradictory requirements of large field-of-view and high spatial resolution. In an effort to maximize both parameters at the same time, a partial field-of-view (pFOV) or focus field coils have been introduced, however at the price of reduced field homogeneity and increased complexity of the apparatus. Here we propose and carry out simulations of a new robust design of field-free line selection coils that also act as focus coils for pFOV MPI scanner.

Experimental Validation of the Selection Field of a Rabbit Sized FFL Scanner

A. Bakenecker[*], T. Friedrich, A. von Gladiß, M. Graeser, J. Stelzner, T. M. Buzug

Institute of Medical Engineering, Universität zu Lübeck, Lübeck, Germany
*Corresponding author, email: {bakenecker,buzug}@imt.uni-luebeck.de

There are two different field topologies in magnetic particle imaging which enable the spatial encoding of the signal. Scanners using a field-free line (FFL) are promising regarding their sensitivity, because the low field volume is larger compared to a field-free point (FFP) and therefore, more particles contribute to the signal. A rabbit-sized FFL scanner with a bore diameter of 173 mm was presented in 2014. After planning and assembling the scanner an experimental validation of the designated field topology of the selection field is presented. With a hall probe the field topologies of the z-gradient coil and the two quadrupoles forming together the selection field of the scanner were investigated. These magnetic field measurements show the expected field topologies: an FFP formed by the z-gradient coil and an FFL parallel to the bore of the scanner formed by each quadrupole. From these measurements the field gradients were calculated and approximated towards the designated currents. The results are in good agreement with the expected field gradients. In order to determine the best suitable frequency for rotating the FFL measurements were done on the power loss in the shielding taking place for higher frequencies. And the power transmission of the transformer, which is problematic for low frequencies. A rotation frequency of 20 Hz is chosen as it represents a compromise between transformer performance and power loss in the shielding.

Spectral Measurements Inside a Rabbit Sized FFL-MPI Device Using a Gradiometric Receive Coil

J. Stelzner[*], M. Graeser, A. Bakenecker, T. M. Buzug

Institute of Medical Engineering, Universität zu Lübeck, Lübeck, Germany
*Corresponding author, email: {stelzner,buzug}@imt.uni-luebeck.de

This work continues prior investigations on the currently world's largest field-free line (FFL) magnetic particle imaging (MPI) scanner. The bore of the imaging device provides a diameter of 173 mm and could accommodate measurement objects like a rabbit. It has already been shown that the drive-field coils capable of conducting an alternating current with a frequency of 25 kHz and an amplitude of slightly above 500 A. With this current input, the drive-field generator produces a magnetic flux density of up to more than 20 mT amplitude in the center of the bore. As the associated magnetic field strength is already sufficient to excite superparamagnetic iron oxide nanoparticles (SPIONs), this work presents an approach to further increase the sensitivity of the system by testing a gradiometric receive coil arrangement.

Differential magnetometry to detect sentinel lymph nodes in laparoscopic procedures

M. van de Loosdrecht[*], S. Waanders, R. Wildeboer, E. Krooshoop, B. ten Haken

MIRA Institute for Biomedical Technology and Technical Medicine, University of Twente, Enschede, Netherlands
*Corresponding author, email: m.m.vandeloosdrecht@utwente.nl

Detection of the sentinel lymph node (SLN) in cancer patients can overrule the requirement for resection of all regional lymph nodes, which leads to decreased morbidity. However, SLN biopsies are currently only clinical practice in breast cancer and melanoma. In other cancer types such as colon cancer, SLNs are located deeper inside the body and therefore the resection procedure is more complicated. A trend that is observed in the medical world is the increased use of minimal invasive interventions. This will in many situations overrule open surgery, which leads to decreased risks to the patient.

The use of magnetic nanoparticles has many advantages over nuclear tracers, which are the current standard to detect SLNs. The principle that we use to achieve SLN detection is differential magnetometry (DiffMag). In DiffMag the nonlinear magnetization characteristics of superparamagnetic iron oxide nanoparticles are exploited. The main drawback of the current handheld Diffmag device is limited depth sensitivity. In order to alleviate this drawback we propose a set-up in which the excitation and detection coils are mechanically separated. As a result, the size of the excitation coil can be increased and placed outside the body. The detection probe can be made much smaller. Our goal is to place the detector inside laparoscopic equipment in order to provide a minimal invasive way to detect SLNs.

Real-time Reconstruction for (TW)MPI Systems

P. Vogel[*, a,b], S. Herz[b], T. Kampf[a,c], M. A. Rückert[a], T. A. Bley[b], V. C. Behr[a]

a) Department of Experimental Physics 5 (Biophysics), University of Würzburg, Würzburg, Germany
b) Department of Diagnostic and Interventional Radiology, University Hospital Würzburg, Würzburg, Germany
c) Department of Diagnostic and Interventional Neuroradiology, University Hospital Würzburg, Würzburg, Germany
*Corresponding author, email: Patrick.Vogel@physik.uni-wuerzburg.de

In the last decade main focusses of the research in the MPI community was mainly hardware development as well as the optimization of reconstruction quality. These steps were essential for improving the MPI technology and bring them into a pre-clinical state.

However, a further important part is the software package working behind such a system, which supports important features for clinical routine and research and has to keep up with state of the art scanner capabilities like adjustable scanning trajectories as well as multiple reconstruction methods. Especially a real-time reconstruction feature is important to use the full potential of the fast imaging capabilities of modern MPI scanners.

In this work a software package is introduced, which allows reconstruction of (TW)MPI data with different reconstruction methods in real-time.

Initial results on 2D mobility MPI

C. Kuhlmann*, T. Viereck, S. Draack, M. Schilling, F. Ludwig

Institut für Elektrische Messtechnik und Grundlagen der Elektrotechnik, TU Braunschweig,
Braunschweig, Germany
*Corresponding author, email: c.kuhlmann@tu-bs.d

Magnetic particle imaging (MPI), being both quantitative and tracer based,
opens the possibility of spatially resolved functional imaging through the
exploitation of changed tracer behavior in dependence on the functional
information to be extracted. Brownian relaxation, as an intrinsic property of
many MPI tracers, offers access to the mobility state of the tracer particles,
and therefore allows spatially resolved mobility MPI (mMPI) imaging.
Through functionalization of particle shells, mobility information can be
varied, e.g. by antibody-antigen binding reactions, allowing functional
imaging with many applications. In order to extract spatial mobility
information and spatial distribution of particles at the same time, we have
built a 2D dual frequency MPI scanner. The additional information gained by
using a second set of drive field frequencies improves sensitivity and contrast
of mMPI with respect to particle mobility. We performed 2D and dual-
frequency MPI scans and evaluated reconstruction by using simulated data.

A report on instrumentation development for magnetic nanoparticles tomography at Nuclear and Medical Electronics Division of Warsaw University of Technology

P. Wróblewski[*], D. Wanta, J. Kryszyn, M. Stosio, W. T. Smolik

Institute of Radioelectronic and Multimedia Technology, Nuclear and Medical Electronics Division, Warsaw university of technology, Warsaw, Poland
*Corresponding author, email: p.wroblewski@stud.elka.pw.edu.pl

This article summarizes all accomplishments of Nuclear and Medical Electronics Division in the field of Magnetic Nanoparticles Imaging, describes most interesting features of developed equipment, as well as reports about research conducted in the Division in prospect of advancement of this imaging method in Poland. Nuclear and Medical Electronics Division of Warsaw University of Technology conduct research on the detectors and data acquisition systems for medical imaging devices. In 2011 the research on instrumentation for magnetic particle imaging was started. In the wake of previous studies, conducted under statutory works, one dimensional nanoparticles scanner was created. Presently system for nanoparticles spectroscopy is being developed. Furthermore, numerical calculation MATLAB toolbox is being written that will allow simulation of MPI measurement system, generation of simulated measurement result of such systems and reconstruction of MPI images from both artificial and real data. Past results motivate us to continue work in this field. Probable next step will be extension of functionality of current MPI scanner model to 2D or 3D imaging, which in turn will allow further research in this new imaging technique.

Poster Session
Methodology

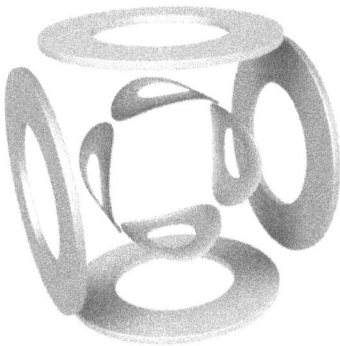

Effect of Core Size Distribution of Immobilized Magnetic Nanoparticles on Harmonic Magnetization

T. Yoshida[*], T. Sasayama, K. Enpuku

Department of Electrical Engineering, Kyushu University, Fukuoka, Japan
*Corresponding author, email: t_yoshi@ees.kyushu-u.ac.jp

In magnetic particle imaging (MPI), harmonic magnetization signals detected from magnetic nanoparticles (MNPs) are used to image the spatial distribution of the MNPs. The strength of the harmonic signals is directly related to the sensitivity of the MPI system. In this study, we used numerical simulations based on the Fokker-Planck equation to explore the effect of the core size distribution of an immobilized MNP sample on the harmonic signals. We assumed an anisotropy value of 5 kJ/m^3 and a uniform volume-weighted core size distribution of MNPs ranging from 17.4 to 37.6 nm to simulate a typical MNPs sample. First, we show that the strength of the harmonic signals of the MNP sample were much lower than calculated from the scalar summation of the harmonic signals generated from each MNP in the sample. For example, the strength of the 9th harmonic signal decreased to one-third. This indicates that about 67 % of the 9th harmonic signals generated from each MNP are mutually cancelled. We then show that the phase lag of the magnetization due to a finite Néel relaxation time caused lower harmonic magnetization signals of the MNP sample when the core size was distributed. These results indicate that an MNP sample with a narrow size distribution and small anisotropy energy would effectively improve the sensitivity of the MPI system.

Remote detection of magnetic signals with compact atomic magnetometer modules towards a MRI-MPI hybrid system

K. Kato, T. Oida, Y. Ito, T. Kobayashi[*]

Graduate School of Engineering, Kyoto University, Kyoto, Japan
*Corresponding author, email: kobayashi.tetsuo.2c@kyoto-u.ac.jp

Optically pumped atomic magnetometers (OPAMs) are based on the detection of electron spin precession in alkali-metal atoms contained in glass cells. In recent years, OPAMs operating under spin-exchange relaxation-free (SERF) conditions have reached sensitivities comparable to and even surpassing those of superconducting quantum interference devices (SQUIDs). In addition, OPAMs have the intrinsic advantage of not requiring cryogenic cooling. Therefore, OPAMs are currently expected to overtake SQUIDs and the possibilities for using OPAMs for biomagnetic field measurements and MRI have been demonstrated. We have been developing a compact and portable OPAM module with a pump-probe arrangement. The noise spectrum density of the OPAM module reached 20 fT/Hz$^{1/2}$ at frequency range of less than 10 kHz. Since sensitivity of OPAM does not depend on frequency, it is suitable to be used as a receiving sensor for magnetic particle imaging (MPI) and ultra-low field-MRI systems. In this study, we demonstrate the possibility to detect magnetic fields generated from magnetic particles (Resovist) and MR signals with a compact OPAM module remotely by using flux transformer towards MRI-MPI hybrid systems. The applicability of new optical MRI-MPI hybrid systems might provide important advancements in neuroscience, neural engineering and improve the clinical diagnosis and management of neurological and psychiatric disorders.

Improvement of Detection Sensitivity for MPI System Based on Vibrating Particles

S. Urushibata[* a], T. Takagi[b], T. Hatsuda[b], A. Matsuhisa[b], M. Arayama[b], Y. Ishihara[a]

a) School of Science and Technology, Meiji University, Japan
b) Graduate School of Science and Technology, Meiji University, Japan
*Corresponding author, email: instrumentation.urushibata@gmail.com

Conventional magnetic particle imaging (MPI) requires generating a gradient magnetic field and an alternative magnetic field. However, when the gradient magnetic field is not sufficiently steep, image artifacts and blurring occur because the magnetization signals are generated from a magnetic nanoparticle (MNP) at even vicinity of a field free point (FFP). Therefore, large coils and multiple power supplies are required to generate the steep gradient magnetic field and the alternative magnetic field. We have proposed a signal detection method by vibrating the MNP without using a large hardware system. Another advantage is that this method can detect the signals with high sensitivity based on the primary harmonic component. A numerical analysis and a phantom experiment were performed to confirm the validity of this proposed method. The results indicated an improvement in the signal-to-noise ratio of the images reconstructed using the proposed method when compared to the conventional signal detection method.

Evaluation of Magnetic Field Strength for FFP line-scanning driven with low electric currents

A. Kuzuhara [a], T. Hatsuda [b], T. Takagi [b], S. Takahashi [b],
M. Arayama [b], Y. Ishihara [a]

a) School of Science and Technology, Meiji University, Japan
b) Graduate School of Science and Technology, Meiji University, Japan
Corresponding author, email: aroof.tantan@gmail.com

Magnetic particle imaging (MPI) has been proposed as a new medical imaging technology, and various systems and image reconstruction methods have been reported. We have constructed a 2-D MPI system with coils driven by relatively low electric currents. However, in this system, a sufficient alternating magnetic field intensity and scanning speed cannot be obtained. Currently, we are attempting to achieve high-speed diagnostic imaging using field-free point (FFP) line scanning, and evaluate the quality of reconstructed images using inverse-problem and iterative reconstruction methods in the proposed system. In this study, we have focused on the alternating magnetic field strength for FFP line scanning to obtain the reconstructed image at high resolution and speed; we also evaluated the alternating magnetic field strength that is necessary for the system.

A Trajectory Study for Obtaining MPI System Matrices in a Compressed-Sensing Framework

M. Maaß[* a)], M. Ahlborg[b)], A. Bakenecker[b)], F. Katzberg[a)],
H. Phan[a)], T. M. Buzug[b)], A. Mertins[a)]

a) Institute for Signal Processing, Universität zu Lübeck, Lübeck, Germany
b) Institute of Medical Engineering, Universität zu Lübeck, Lübeck, Germany
*Corresponding author, email: maass@isip.uni-luebeck.de

In this paper, we study the efficiency of five different field free point trajectories in two-dimensional magnetic particle imaging for the compressed-sensing based reconstruction of partially measured system matrices. To show the suitability of the trajectories, different trajectories with identical repetition times were simulated using on the same scanner setup. We show that for all trajectories, the compressed-sensing based reconstruction approach for the system matrix is possible and promising for real-world scenarios. Also we validate the already known fact that the Lissajous trajectory is appropriate for the compressed sensing approach. However, there are still other trajectory choices which show similar and even better performance in the compressed-sensing based reconstruction.

Poster Session

Tracer Materials

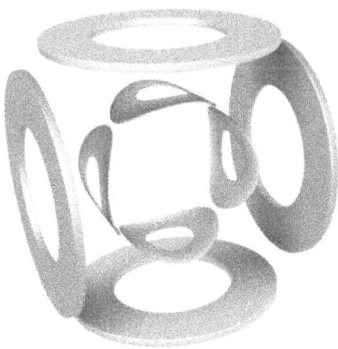

MPS and MRI efficacy of magnetosomes from wild-type and mutant bacterial strains

D. Heinke[* a], A. Kraupner[a], D. Eberbeck[b], D. Schmidt[b], R. Uebe[b], D. Schüler[c], A. Briel[a]

a) nanoPET Pharma GmbH, Berlin, Germany
b) Physikalisch-Technische Bundesanstalt, Berlin, Germany
c) University of Bayreuth, Bayreuth, Germany
*Corresponding author, email: david.heinke@nanopet.de

The future of Magnetic Particle Imaging (MPI), as a tracer-based imaging modality, crucially relies on the development of high-performing tracers. Due to their ideal structural and magnetic properties, biogenic nanoparticles extracted from magnetotactic bacteria are promising candidates for MPI tracer research. In the present study we investigate the potential of bacterial magnetosomes, extracted from wild-type bacteria of the strain Magnetospirillum gryphiswaldense and various mutants thereof, as new tracer materials for MPI. Furthermore, we investigate the structural and magnetic properties of the magnetosomes as well as their suitability as Magnetic Resonance Imaging (MRI) agents in order to explain differences in MPI and MRI efficacies.

Synthesis and Characterisation of Superparamagnetic Polylactic acid based Polymers

C. Jacobi, K. Lüdtke-Buzug[*]

Institute of Medical Engineering, Universität zu Lübeck, Lübeck, Germany
*Corresponding author, email: luedtke-buzug@imt.uni-luebeck.de

In this article, a novel superparamagnetic polymer is introduced for the use in magnetic particle imaging (MPI). This MPI-sensitive material is synthesized by the addition of superparamagnetic iron-oxide nanoparticles (SPIONs) during the last step of the synthesis chain of the chosen polymer, that is in the case discussed here, polylactic acid (PLA). The synthesis products are characterized by magnetic particle spectrometry (MPS) as a utility indicator for MPI, because a strong signal in the harmonics of the signal spectrum is a necessary condition for visibility in MPI. We demonstrate experimentally that the produced compound is MPI-visible. A stable and biocompatible polymer material that gives contrast in MPI opens the door to many medical procedures, for instance, surgical devices may be coated with superparamagnetic PLA and then tracked with magnetic-based navigation instruments. Furthermore, stents and catheters may be coated with PLA, which would allow their navigation inside the vascular system, eliminating today's radiation dose in the catheter lab.

Resolution study on new MPI tracer material

C. Debbeler[*], K. Lüdtke-Buzug

Institute of Medical Engineering, Universität zu Lübeck, Lübeck, Germany
*Corresponding author, email: {debbeler,luedtke-buzug}@imt.uni-luebeck.de

With the progressive development of Magnetic Particle Imaging (MPI), the research on suitable tracer materials gains importance as well. In the scope of the EU financed NanoMag project, which objectives are the standardization, improvement and redefinition of manufacturing technologies as well as analyzing methods, newly synthesized magnetic nanoparticles (MNPs) are investigated regarding their suitability as MPI tracers using Magnetic Particle Spectroscopy (MPS) and MPI. Two MNP samples synthesized by nanoPET Pharma GmbH and one MNP sample from the Department of Physics of the Technical University of Denmark were investigated using the MPS system and a preclinical MPI scanner located in Lübeck. First measurements in both systems show that the performance of all three samples is comparable to the one of Resovist, which is currently known as a gold standard MPI tracer. In a next step, the suitability of those three samples as well as several other available MNP samples will be investigated in a resolution study in order to further analyze the achievable sensitivity and spatial resolution of the particles.

Linearized spectra of Preclinical MPI scanner for tracer characterization

O. Kosch[* a)], J. Franke[b)], G. Bringout[a)], N. Löwa[a)], L. Trahms[a)], F. Wiekhorst[a)]

a) Physikalisch-Technische Bundesanstalt, Berlin, Germany
b) Bruker Biospin MRI GmbH, Ettlingen, Germany
*Corresponding author, email: olaf.kosch@ptb.de

We investigated the spectra obtained by Magnetic Particle Spectroscopy (MPS) and Magnetic Particle Imaging (MPI) of different magnetic Nanoparticles (Resovist, fluidMAG-D, HK) to identify spectral components appropriate for image reconstruction by MPI. The MPS spectra allowed the estimation of the particular amplitudes resolvable by MPI for the different considered MNP types. Then, we measured the transfer function of the Berlin preclinical MPI-scanner to linearize the MPI spectra. For MPI measurement and image reconstruction the analysis of noise level and the reduction related to the tracer signal are the main issues. With regard to image reconstruction of a rectangular phantom (1 cm x 1cm x 0.5 cm) filled with MNP, we found that values of the highest frequencies with a sufficient signal-to-noise-ratio determine the reconstruction quality. By applying this to the spectra of the MPI-scanner, we were able to characterize rapidly a magnetic tracer with regard to MPI imaging properties without having to measure a time consuming system function.

Magnetic Particle Spectrometry of Fe3O4 nanoclustered particles

L. Abelmann[*], M. Ledwig, L. Pan, B. C. Park, Y. K. Kim

Korea Institute of Science and Technology Europe, Saarbrücken, Germany
*Corresponding author, email: L.Abelmann@kist-europe.de

In this contribution we investigate whether nanoclusters of 10 nm sized Fe3O4 granules with total sizes ranging from 33 to 120 nm would be suitable for magnetic particle imaging. The physical and hydrodynamic radius were measured, as well as the zeta potential. The magnetic response to quasi-static and 20 kHz alternating fields were measured, and compared to a standard FeraSpin R solution. Compared to the other nanoclusters, those of 48 nm average diameter show a much higher dynamic radius, a strong dependence on the applied field and a very straight harmonic phase relation.

Session III
Methodology I

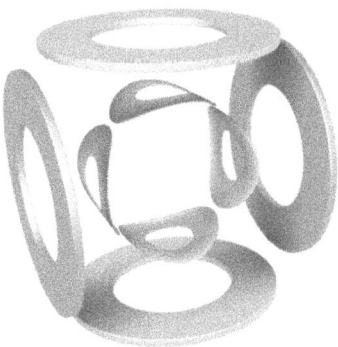

SNR and Discretization Enhancement for System Matrix Determination by Decreasing the Gradient in Magnetic Particle Imaging

M. Graeser[*], A. von Gladiß, T. Friedrich, T. M. Buzug

Institute of Medical Engineering, Universität zu Lübeck, Lübeck, Germany
*Corresponding author, email: {graeser,buzug}@imt.uni-luebeck.de

In system matrix (SM) based reconstruction, the physical resolution is often within the range of the SM discretization. This is caused by the signal to noise ratio (SNR) decrease following a discretization increase due to the smaller particle sample volume. As the SNR affects the resolution of the image as well, it is necessary to decouple the SNR and discretization. In this work, a calibration protocol is presented which enhances either the SNR or discretization by reducing the gradient strength within the system calibration. This new protocol results in higher resolution and better image quality.

Applying Compressed Sensing on Hybrid System Matrices in Magnetic Particle Imaging

A. von Gladiß[*], M. Graeser, T. M. Buzug

Institute of Medical Engineering, Universität zu Lübeck, Lübeck, Germany
*Corresponding author, email: {gladiss,buzug}@imt.uni-luebeck.de

Reconstruction in Magnetic Particle Imaging can be performed using a system matrix that encodes the spectral response of the system to a delta sample at different spatial positions of the field of view. The system matrix is acquired prior to the measurement in a time-consuming process.

Compressed sensing has successfully been applied to the acquisition scheme of system matrices in order to reduce the measurement time. Recently, it has been shown that hybrid system matrices that are acquired in a dedicated device can be used for reconstructing images in Magnetic Particle Imaging. They are superior to device-own system matrices in terms of signal to noise ratio and measurement time. In this work, compressed sensing is applied to hybrid system matrices.

Model uncertainty in magnetic particle imaging: Motivating nonlinear problems by model-based sparse reconstruction

T. Kluth[*], P. Maass

Center for Industrial Mathematics, University of Bremen, Bremen
*Corresponding author, email: tkluth@math.uni-bremen.de

In magnetic particle imaging the concentration of superparamagnetic iron oxide nanoparticles is determined by measuring the particle's nonlinear response to an applied magnetic field. The particles are highly sensitive to the dynamic magnetic field which allows a rapid data acquisition. As a result magnetic particle imaging benefits from a high temporal resolution and can reach high spatial resolutions. But model-based reconstruction techniques are still not able to reach the quality of data-based approaches. In the latter case the linear system function is determined by a time-consuming measurement process which also has negative implications for the spatial resolution of the reconstructions. Common model approaches are overly simplified leading to reconstructions of minor quality. Possible reasons for insufficient reconstructions include the behavior of nanoparticles in fast changing magnetic fields. For example, the simple model of paramagnetism described by the Langevin function is not sufficient to describe potentially emerging relaxation effects. We aim for the formulation of nonlinear parameter identification problems which are able to deal with possible model errors while reconstructing a sparse concentration. For this purpose we investigate the commonly used model-based approach with respect to simplifying assumptions and derive the formal definition of the problem. Sparsity constraints are introduced for the concentration function and data-based as well as model-based reconstructions are computed from publicly available data. Finally, nonlinear problems for future research are formulated based on the previous theoretical and numerical investigations.

Improved image reconstruction in magnetic particle imaging using structural a priori information

C. Bathke[* a)], T. Kluth[a)], C. Brandt[b)], P. Maass[a)]

a) Center for Industrial Mathematics, University of Bremen, Bremen, Germany
b) Department of Applied Physics, University of Eastern Finland, Kuopio, Finland
*Corresponding author, email: cbathke@math.uni-bremen.de

Magnetic particle imaging is a tracer-based imaging modality developed to detect the concentration of superparamagnetic iron oxide nanoparticles. The capability for imaging is due to the high sensitivity to the nanoparticle's nonlinear response to the applied magnetic field. This modality relies on the spatial distribution of the tracer material which makes it suitable for applications such as imaging blood flow or tracking medical instruments without the need of harmful radiation. Magnetic particle imaging benefits from a high temporal resolution, but it also suffers from missing background information, e.g., from biological tissue. Commonly the lack of information is remedied by magnetic resonance imaging. Image reconstructions from both modalities are computed independently and aligned subsequently to allow inferences. We use the additional information commonly provided by magnetic resonance imaging to improve the reconstruction in magnetic particle imaging. For this purpose, a Tikhonov-type functional is equipped with a structural prior where the additional information is incorporated. By minimizing this functional, we obtain improved reconstructions of the concentration of nanoparticles which is illustrated in numerical simulations.

Comparison of System-Matrix-Based and Projection-Based Reconstructions for Field Free Line Magnetic Particle Imaging

S. Ilbey[* a], C. B. Top[a], A. Güngör[a], T. Cukur[b,c], E. U. Saritas[b,c], H. E. Güven[a]

a) Advanced Sensing Research Program Department, ASELSAN A. Ş., Turkey
b) Department of Electrical and Electronics Engineering, Bilkent University, Ankara, Turkey
c) National Magnetic Resonance Research Center (UMRAM), Bilkent University, Ankara, Turkey
*Corresponding author, email: silbey@aselsan.com.tr

In magnetic particle imaging (MPI), system sensitivity can be enhanced by scanning the sample along a field free line (FFL) instead of a field free point (FFP). FFL MPI data can then be processed via system-matrix or projection-based reconstructions. Here, we compare the relative performance of these two approaches. We assume an ideal FFL (straight and homogeneous), which is translated and rotated in a two-dimensional field-of-view. We simulate the acquired data from a numerical vessel phantom for a broad range of noise levels. For the system-matrix reconstruction, we propose Alternating Direction Method of Multipliers (ADMM) to solve a constrained convex optimization problem. We also analyze the results of the nonnegative fused lasso (NFL) model to compare the performance of ADMM with one of the state-of-the-art system matrix based methods. For the projection-based reconstruction, we use the inverse Radon transform formulation with x-space reconstruction. Although all methods yield visibly high quality reconstructions, ADMM produces images with improved structural similarity index at relatively high signal-to-noise-ratios compared to NFL and x-space reconstruction methods. Moreover, ADMM results have lower normalized root-mean-square error at all noise levels.

Session IV

Methodology II

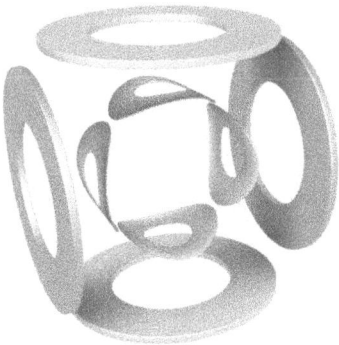

Influence of Orthogonal Receive Channels on the Spatial Resolution in Magnetic Particle Imaging

P. Szwargulski* a,b), T. Knopp a,b)

a) Section for Biomedical Imaging, University Medical Center Hamburg-Eppendorf, Hamburg, Germany
b) Institute for Biomedical Imaging, Hamburg University of Technology, Hamburg, Germany
*Corresponding author, email: p.szwargulski@uke.de

Magnetic Particle Imaging (MPI) is a fast and highly sensitive tomographic imaging modality. When applying 3D Lissajous imaging sequences, the region of interest is rapidly sampled by moving a field-free point along a predefined trajectory. Since the field excitation is done using three orthogonal excitation coils, usually also the magnetization response is measured with three independent and orthogonal receive coils. In this work the influence of selecting a subset of receive channels during reconstruction on the resulting image quality is analyzed. It is shown that using a single receive channel a slight loss of spatial resolution in the order of 12–22 % in the direction perpendicular to the receiving direction can be observed while in direction of the receive coil the resolution is preserved and partially even improved. Since the construction of decoupled 3D receive coil units is a major engineering effort, the findings can be used to simplify the construction of 3D Lissajous type scanners.

Improving the Spatial Resolution of Bidirectional Cartesian MPI Data using Fourier Techniques

F. Werner[* a,b)], N. Gdaniec [a,b)], T. Knopp [a,b)]

a) Section for Biomedical Imaging, University Medical Center Hamburg-Eppendorf, Germany
b) Institute for Biomedical Imaging, University of Technology Hamburg, Germany
*Corresponding author, email: f.werner@uke.de

Magnetic Particle Imaging (MPI) determines the distribution of superparamagnetic nanoparticles. Signal encoding is achieved by moving a field-free point (FFP) through the volume of interest. Due to its simplicity the Cartesian trajectory is used in many experimental scanner setups. One drawback of the Cartesian trajectory is that the spatial resolution is anisotropic and in particular lower in the orthogonal excitation direction. In order to get fully isotropic resolution one can extend the unidirectional Cartesian trajectory to a bidirectional Cartesian trajectory that switches the excitation direction after a first pass over the volume of interest. When reconstructing each of the unidirectional datasets using e.g. an analytical x-space approach, one obtains two images each having a higher spatial resolution in the excitation direction. Within this work, we introduce a postprocessing method that combines both images and calculates a combined image with fully isotropic spatial resolution.

Selective Signal Suppression in MPI: Focusing on Areas of high Signal Intensity Range

S. Herz[* a], P. Vogel[a,b], T. Kampf[b,c], M. A. Rückert[b], V. C. Behr[b], T. A. Bley[a]

a) Department of Diagnostic and Interventional Radiology, University Hospital Würzburg, Würzburg, Germany
b) Department of Experimental Physics 5 (Biophysics), University of Würzburg, Würzburg, Germany
c) Department of Diagnostic and Interventional Neuroradiology, University Hospital Würzburg, Würzburg, Germany
*Corresponding author, email: Herz_S@ukw.de

Introduction: Common MPI scanners have difficulties to correctly visualize areas with a broad signal intensity spectrum due to their low signal dynamic capability. The aim of this study was to develop a selective signal suppression technique using an advanced trajectory design to circumvent this issue.

Materials and Methods: Simulations where performed for a traveling wave (TW) MPI scanner. In the so called slice-scanning mode the field free points (FFPs) travel through the scanner on a sinusoidal trajectory given by the frequencies of the dynamic linear gradient array and a perpendicular saddle coil system. The signal can be selectively suppressed by locally reducing the speed of the FFPs. Series of measurements with two point samples containing different SPIO concentrations with and without selective signal suppression technique were simulated.

Results: When imaging samples with two markedly different SPIO concentrations in the slice-scanning mode the signal of the lower concentration cannot be properly reconstructed. Applying the signal suppression technique to the area of the high concentration sample selectively reduces this signal and demarcates samples with lower concentrations.

Conclusion: A selective signal suppression technique for TWMPI is introduced which allows to focus on low SPIO concentrations in samples with a large range of tracer concentrations. This can facilitate preclinical functional imaging in the proximity of organs with high unspecific SPIO uptake such as the liver.

Artifact Analysis for Axially Elongated Lissajous Trajectories in Magnetic Particle Imaging

C. Kaethner[*], A. Haensch, A. Cordes, T. M. Buzug

Institute of Medical Engineering, Universität zu Lübeck, Lübeck, Germany
*Corresponding author, email: {Kaethner,buzug}@imt.uni-luebeck.de

Magnetic Particle Imaging promises great potential for various imaging scenarios with medical purpose. In order to meet this potential, one of the key factors is that the size and the shape of the sampling area need to be adaptable to the aimed applications. An interesting approach to achieve this within medical and technical safety limits is by use of focus fields. However, even with current focus-field approaches, an enlargement in axial direction remains a challenging task. Recently, a use of an elongated sampling trajectory was proposed to address this challenge. Such an elongation can be achieved either by superimposing an orthogonal oriented linear focus field to a 2D trajectory or by an additional continuous movement in axial direction. The resulting elongated trajectory allows for a larger axial coverage of a scanned object. However, based on the physical properties of the signal generation, the elongation length needs to be limited to avoid signal loss or the occurrence of artifacts. In this work, a simulation based artifact analysis is carried out for Lissajous trajectories to determine an elongation limit that allows for both, the avoidance of signal loss and artifacts.

Submillimeter Accurate Marker Localization within Low Gradient Magnetic Particle Imaging Tomograms

F. Griese [a], T. Knopp [a], R. Werner [b], A. Schlaefer [c], M. Möddel [a]

a) Section for Biomedical Imaging, University Medical Center Hamburg, Hamburg, Germany
b) Section for Image Processing and Medical Informatics, University Medical Center Hamburg, Hamburg, Germany
c) Institute of Medical Technology, Hamburg University of Technology, Germany
*Corresponding author, email: m.hofmann@uke.de

Magnetic Particle Imaging (MPI) achieves a high temporal resolution, which opens up a wide range of real-time medical applications such as device tracking and navigation. These applications usually rely on automated techniques for finding and localizing devices and fiducial markers in medical images. In this work, we show that submillimeter-accurate automatic marker localization from low gradient MPI tomograms with a spatial resolution of several millimeters is possible. Markers are initially identified within the tomograms by a thresholding-based segmentation algorithm. Subsequently, their positions are accurately determined by calculating the center of mass of the gray values inside the pre-segmented regions. A series of phantom measurements taken at full temporal resolution (46 Hz) is used to analyze statistical and systematical errors and to discuss the performance and stability of the automatic submillimeter-accurate marker localization algorithm.

Keynote 2

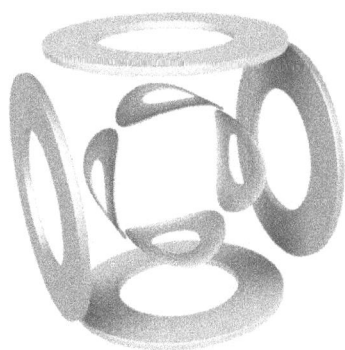

In vivo behavior of SPION and how to modify their destiny

Mauro Magnani

Department of Biomolecular Sciences, University of Urbino and EryDel SpA, Italy

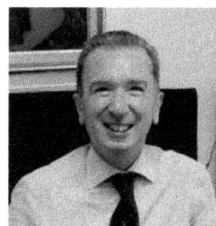

SPIO contrasting agents have been originally approved to improve the sensitivity and the detection of lesions or organ architecture by Magnetic Resonance Imaging (MRI). However, innovative delivery systems able to prolong SPION residence time in the bloodstream, could be very useful in moving forward functional cardiovascular diagnosis and therapeutic monitoring.

Among the several proposed approaches, strategies based on the use of red blood cells (RBCs) as SPION biomimetic carriers useful in diagnostic applications of the vascular system have been suggested. Encapsulation of SPIOs into RBCs appears the most attractive strategy to combine blood resident time with resolution and sensitivity in MRI and MPI.

During the years we have developed a procedure for the safe encapsulation of SPIO nanoparticles, such as Resovist®, Sinerem, Endorem, P904 and Ferucarbotran, into RBCs, documented that these constructs are stable in vitro and in vivo and that can prolong the circulation time of these contrasting agents.

The results obtained in vivo, in the mouse, have showed that it is possible to prolong the half-life of iron-based contrasting agents changing the destiny of bulk nanoparticles that otherwise would be rapidly cleared in few minutes. Several additional approaches permit to reduce or extent the half-life in circulation and both PK and PD of SPION.

Session V
Methodology III

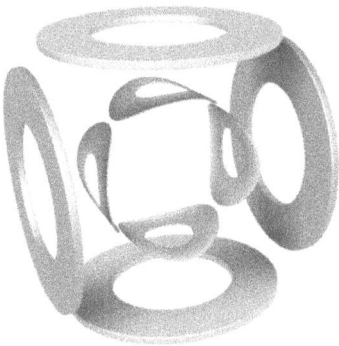

Multifunctional SPIONs for Theranostics in Cancer

S. Lyer[* a)], T. Knopp[b)], F. Werner[b)], J. Zaloga[a)], R. Friedrich[a)],
F. Wiekhorst[c)], T. Struffert[d)], T. Engelhorn[d)], A. Dörfler[d)],
T. Bäuerle[d)], M. Uder[d)], R. Tietze[a)], C. Janko[a)], C. Alexiou[a)]

a) Universitätsklinikum Erlangen, Department of Otorhinolaryngology, Head and Neck Surgery, Section of Experimental Oncology and Nanomedicine, Erlangen, Germany
b) Universitätsklinikum Hamburg-Eppendorf, Diagnostic and Interventional Radiology Department and Clinic, Hamburg, Germany
c) Physikalisch Technische Bundesanstalt, Berlin, Germany
d) Universitätsklinikum Erlangen, Department of Radiology/Neuroradiology, Erlangen, Germany
*Corresponding author, email: stefan.lyer@uk-erlangen.de

Due to their magnetic properties, superparamagnetic iron oxide nanoparticles (SPIONs) offer a large variety of possibilities for medical applications. In Magnetic Particle Imaging (MPI) to date SPIONs are the only tracers or imaging agents so far. It is proposed that the optimal tracer for MPI is a single core SPION with a core diameter of around 30 nm. However, such particles seem not to be optimal for magnetically enhanced drug delivery. On the other hand, there are multicore particles equipped with a high loading capacity for drugs, which can be accumulated e.g. in a tumor by a static magnetic field and additionally be heated by an alternating magnetic field. Here we show that such particles cannot be only imaged by magnetic resonance imaging (MRI) but also do show a MPI-signal. Providing, that the sensitivity of MPI for such particles and therefore also the resolution is high enough, this could be exploited to estimate the SPION-mediated drug load in a tumor after Magnetic Drug Targeting (MDT) as a real theranostic approach.

Magnetic nanoparticle temperature imaging with a 2D magnetic particle spectrometer scanner

J. Zhong[*], F. Ludwig, M. Schilling

Institut für Elektrische Messtechnik und Grundlagen der Elektrotechnik, TU Braunschweig, Germany
*Corresponding author, email: j.zhong@tu-braunschweig.de

This study reports on 2D magnetic nanoparticle (MNP) temperature imaging with a 2D magnetic particle spectrometer scanner. A mechanical scanner is redesigned to measure the MNP harmonics whereas a reconstruction method based on the point spread function of a pick-up coil is proposed to reconstruct the MNP temperature. Phantom experiments demonstrate the feasibility of the proposed method for temperature imaging.

Temperature-dependent MPS measurements

S. Draack[*], T. Viereck, C. Kuhlmann, M. Schilling, F. Ludwig

Institut für Elektrische Messtechnik und Grundlagen der Elektrotechnik, TU Braunschweig,
Braunschweig, Germany
*Corresponding author, email: s.draack@tu-bs.de

The non-linear signal generation in Magnetic Particle Imaging (MPI) using
magnetic nanoparticles as tracer materials is still not fully explained and a
far-reaching research area. Magnetic Particle Spectroscopy (MPS) was
developed to investigate the particle behavior in high externally applied
magnetic field strengths and to derive mathematical models which describe
the physical processes in MPI in detail. A new MPS setup was built which
allows measurements between -13 °C and +114 °C in order to investigate the
temperature dependence of the harmonics spectra. Temperature-dependent
MPS measurements of diluted FeraSpinTM XL, either as suspension or
freeze-dried in a mannitol matrix, using the new setup are shown and
exemplarily discussed.

Effects of Duty Cycle on Magnetostimulation Thresholds in MPI

O. B. Demirel[* a,b)], E. U. Saritas [a,b)]

a) Department of Electrical and Electronics Engineering, Bilkent Univeristy, Ankara, Turkey
b) National Magnetic Resonance Research Center (UMRAM), Bilkent University, Ankara, Turkey
*Corresponding author, email: demirel@ee.bilkent.edu.tr

Magnetic Particle Imaging (MPI) relies on time-varying magnetic fields to generate an image of the spatial distribution of superparamagnetic iron oxide nanoparticles. However, these oscillating magnetic field form electric field patterns within the body, which in turn can cause peripheral nerve stimulations (PNS), also known as magnetostimulation. To prevent potential safety hazards and to optimize the scanning parameters such as field-of-view (FOV) and scanning speed in MPI, the factors that affect drive field magnetostimulation limits need to be determined accurately. In this work, we investigate the effects of the duty cycle on magnetostimulation thresholds in MPI. We performed human subject experiments by using a highly homogenous solenoidal coil on the upper arm of six subjects. Six different duty cycles ranging between 5% and 100% were applied at 25 kHz. Accordingly, magnetostimulation limits first decrease and then increase with increasing duty cycle, reaching a maximum at 100% duty cycle. Since high duty cycles would be the preferred operating mode for rapid imaging with MPI, these results have promising implications for future human-sized MPI systems.

Preparing system functions for quantitative MPI

O. Kosch[* a], U. Heinen [b], L. Trahms [a], F. Wiekhorst [a]

a) Department 8.2 Biosignals, Physikalisch-Technische Bundesanstalt, Berlin, Germany
b) Department of Electrical Engineering & Information Technology, University of Applied Sciences, Pforzheim
*Corresponding author, email: olaf.kosch@ptb.de

Theoretically, Magnetic particle imaging (MPI) pledges quantitative imaging of magnetic nanoparticle (MNP) distributions. By an eight-shaped hosepipe phantom experiment using Ferucarbotran (Resovist precursor) as a tracer, we investigated the quantification capability of a commercial preclinical MPI-scanner (Bruker/Philips Preclinical MPI System, Germany) operated at Charité university hospital, Berlin. For reconstruction of MPI images of the MNP distribution we used a set of four system functions (SF) acquired with a tracer reference at different iron concentrations (in the range 0.1 mol/L to 1 mol/L). From the analysis of a selected region of interest in the reconstructed images, we found a linear relation between voxel values and the inverse of the concentration of the corresponding reference used in the particular SF acquisition. Based on the precisely known total tracer amount, we determined the tracer amount of each single voxel volume in the phantom from the MPI image. This could be achieved independent of the concentration of the reference used in the SF acquisition.

Session VI
Instrumentation II

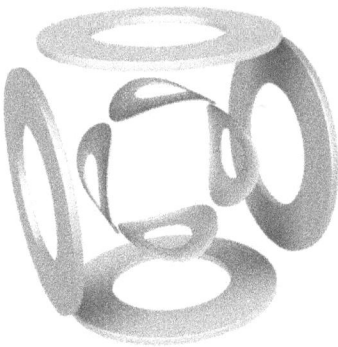

A Magneto Acoustic Spectrometer

T. Friedrich[*], N. Schreiner, T. M. Buzug

Institute of Medical Engineering, Universität zu Lübeck, Lübeck, Germany
*Corresponding author, email: friedrich@imt.uni-luebeck.de

Oscillating magnetic fields may generate vibrations in an object containing magnetic nanoparticles. These vibrations can lead to sound waves traveling through surrounding media like biological tissue. The detection of these sound waves was proposed to enable magneto acoustic elastography, which could be used to gain additional information about the object being scanned in an MPI device. This paper describes the construction of a prototype for a magneto acoustic spectrometer. To demonstrate the spectrometers capabilities, gel phantoms with SPION fillings have been examined and the results are shown.

A summing configuration based Low noise amplifier for MPI and MPS

A. Malhotra[*], T. M. Buzug

Institute of Medical Engineering, Universität zu Lübeck, Lübeck, Germany
*Corresponding author, email: {malhotra,buzug}@imt.uni-luebeck.de

In the current research a low noise amplifier suitable for the Magnetic Particle Imaging and the Magnetic Particle Spectroscopy is presented. LNA plays a significant role in the send chain of the MPI and MPS and can increase the resolution of signal by adding higher harmonics to the spectrum. The LNA is based on the summing configuration and fabricated on a printed circuit board. Moreover, the prototyped LNA is compared with a commercially available pre-amplifier. The input voltage noise of the prototyped LNA is approximately 440 pA/√Hz.

First measured result of the 3D Magnetic Particle Spectrometer

X. Chen[*], M. Graeser, A. Behrends, T. M. Buzug

Institute of Medical Engineering, Universität zu Lübeck, Lübeck, Germany
*Corresponding author, email: {chen,buzug}@imt.uni-luebeck.de

Magnetic Particle Imaging (MPI) is capable of imaging the spatial distribution of superparamagnetic iron oxide (SPIO) nanoparticles with a high sensitivity and high resolution. A Magnetic Particle Spectrometer (MPS) can be used to estimate the magnetic response of the SPIO nanoparticles and achieve the system matrix for the calibration of imaging devices. A one-dimensional and two-dimensional MPS have been introduced and shown good usability. A three-dimensional transmit coil setup was optimized, and its corresponding signal chains have been partially described. This paper is a continuation work and aims at presenting the first measured results of the three-dimensional MPS.

Real-time 3D Dynamic Rotational Slice-Scanning Mode for Traveling Wave MPI

P. Vogel[* a,b)], M. A. Rückert[a)], P. Klauer[a)], S. Herz[b)], T. Kampf[a,c)], T. A. Bley[b)], V. C. Behr[a)]

a) Department of Experimental Physics 5 (Biophysics), University of Würzburg, Würzburg, Germany
b) Department of Diagnostic and Interventional Radiology, University Hospital Würzburg, Würzburg, Germany
c) Department of Diagnostic and Interventional Neuroradiology, University Hospital Würzburg, Würzburg, Germany
*Corresponding author, email: Patrick.Vogel@physik.uni-wuerzburg.de

Magnetic Particle Imaging is a tomographic imaging technique offering a high sensitivity and temporal resolution and is a promising tool for pre-clinical applications. The existing Traveling Wave Magnetic Particle Imaging scanners offer a mouse-sized FOV. Several sequences have been introduced to scan the entire FOV in 3D. Unfortunately, the proposed 3D sequences do not provide real-time capability, which is an important feature for prospected applications in clinical routine.

In this work a modified sequence is presented, which allows scanning an entire 3D volume on a short time scale and offers a 3D visualization in real-time.

Session VII

Applications

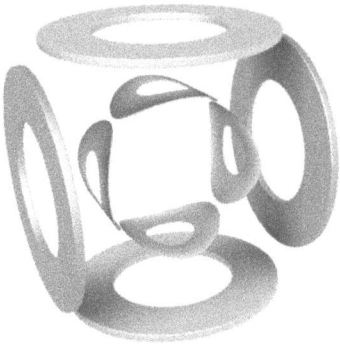

Towards the Integration of a Magnetic Particle Imaging Compatible Ultrasound Transducer

T. C. Kranemann[*], T. Ersepke, G. Schmitz

Chair for Medical Engineering, Ruhr-Universität Bochum, Bochum, Germany
*Corresponding author, email: Tim.Kranemann@rub.de

Magnetic particle imaging (MPI) is a tracer based imaging modality and thus lacks anatomical information. Medical ultrasound (US) imaging might provide real-time morphological data to be combined with functional MPI images. However, a standard US device will possibly be damaged by the strong alternating magnetic fields inside the MPI bore. Moreover, US equipment might degrade the MPI signal quality. In this work, critical US components prone to eddy current heating are pointed out by exemplary presenting the functional groups of a commercial medical US transducer. A theoretical model is utilized to derive maximum applicable sizes for electrode surfaces and transducer cables. Heating experiments confirm the theoretical model and components show no destructive heating when structure sizes are reasonably small. Further, transducer dummies are used to measure the interferences between both modalities. The MPI signals show a minor increase in the noise level when transducer dummies are present, while a significant increase is recognized when transducer dummies are actively driven. The US signals show strong disturbances in the frequency range of the MPI drive fields during MPI acquisition, which is orders of magnitude lower than the relevant US frequency range. It is concluded that the combination of an MPI scanner and an adapted US hardware is possible. Future work needs to address the influence of mutual interferences with regard to the reconstruction algorithms of both modalities.

Magnetic Particle Imaging of liver tumors in small animal models

J. Dieckhoff[* a)], M. G. Kaul[a)], T. Mummert[a)], C. Jung[a)], J. Salamon[a)], G. Adam[a)], T. Knopp[b,c)], D. Schwinge[d)], H. Ittrich[a)]

a) Department for Diagnostic and Interventional Radiology and Nuclear Medicine, University Medical Center Hamburg-Eppendorf, Hamburg, Germany
b) Section for Biomedical Imaging, University Medical Center Hamburg-Eppendorf, Hamburg, Germany
c) Institute for Biomedical Imaging, Hamburg University of Technology, Hamburg, Germany
d) I. Department of Internal Medicine, University Medical Center Hamburg-Eppendorf, Hamburg, Germany
*Corresponding author, email: j.dieckhoff@uke.de

In vivo liver visualization can be realized with Magnetic Particle Imaging (MPI) since a major part of the iron oxide nanoparticles – intravenously injected and imaged with MPI – is finally taken up by the mononuclear phagocytic system (MPS) of the liver. In this study, the possibility to detect and characterize liver tumors with MPI was analyzed. Genetically modified mice developing hepatocellular carcinoma (HCC) were continuously screened with high-field MRI. In case of liver lesions with diameters larger 5 mm, the mice were sequentially imaged with MRI and MPI after the intravenous injection of ferucarbotran (Resovist®). For comparison of liver morphologies represented by MPI and MRI, image data of both modalities were fused assisted by external MPI and MRI fiducial markers. A good correlation between MPI and MRI images was found with image analysis-based 2-D correlation coefficients of around 0.7. Liver lesions – characterized by a missing accumulation of ferucarbotran – led to signal gaps or drops in the MPI signal depending on their actual size and location. While lesions with diameters larger than 5 mm caused visible effects in the MPI signal, smaller sized lesions could not be detected. This was mainly attributed to the comparable low MPI resolution of a few millimeters in this study. The principle feasibility of liver tumor visualizations with MPI was demonstrated motivating more detailed studies on liver MPI for diagnostic and interventional applications.

Detection of flow dynamic change in a 3D printed aneurysm model after treatment

J. Sedlacik[* a)], A. Frölich[a)], J. Spallek[b)], N. D. Forkert[c)],
F. Werner[d,e)], T. Knopp[d,e)], D. Krause[b)], J. Fiehler[a)], J.-H. Buhk[a)]

a) Neuroradiology, University Medical Center Hamburg-Eppendorf, Hamburg, Germany
b) Product Development and Mechanical Engineering Design, Hamburg University of Technology, Hamburg, Germany
c) Department of Radiology and Hotchkiss Brain Institute, University of Calgary, Calgary, AB, Canada
d) Section for Biomedical Imaging, University Medical Center Hamburg-Eppendorf, Hamburg, Germany
e) Institute for Biomedical Imaging, Hamburg University of Technology, Hamburg, Germany
*Corresponding author, email: j.sedlacik@uke.de

Treatment success and potential relapse of intracranial aneurysms need to be followed-up by regular imaging. However, the metallic material inside treated aneurysms can cause artifacts in MRI, CT and DSA possibly compromising clinical interpretation. Furthermore, frequent follow-ups with X-ray based imaging methods seriously increase the patient's exposure to ionizing radiation. Thus, magnetic particle imaging (MPI) may be beneficial for patients with treated aneurysms. The purpose of this work was to demonstrate the capability of MPI to depict the change of the contrast agent dynamics of aneurysms after treatment. Realistic aneurysm models before and after treatment by different means were connected to a peristaltic pump with a physiologic flow (250 ml/min) and pulsation rate (70/min). Contrast agent curves over time were measured during injection of a 3 ml bolus within 3 s of an aqueous solution of 50 mmol(Fe)/L. MPI was able to detect the expected delay and dispersion of the contrast agent in the treated aneurysm as well as a less filling with contrast agent, if densely packed material was present inside the aneurysm. The delay was estimated based on the MPI contrast agent curves to be in the order of about 1 s. Thus, MPI is capable to detect delay and dispersion of the contrast agent dynamics after aneurysm treatment with clinical standard metallic material.

MPI Flow Analysis Toolbox exploiting pulsed tracer information – an aneurysm phantom proof

J. Franke[*][a,b)], R. Lacroix[c)], H. Lehr[a)], M. Heidenreich[a)], U. Heinen[d)],
V. Schulz[b)]

a) Bruker BioSpin MRI GmbH, Ettlingen, Germany
b) Physics of Molecular Imaging Systems, University RWTH Aachen, Germany
c) GE Healthcare, Strategic Development in Advanced Applications, Buc, France
d) University of Applied Sciences Pforzheim, Pforzheim, Germany
*Corresponding author, email: jochen.franke@bruker.com

Assessment of flow parameters provides insight into (patho-)physiology and thus is a common tool in the field of cardiology to screen for or to evaluate and stage cardiovascular diseases. In this work, we present a Flow Analysis Toolbox for Magnetic Particle Imaging datasets highlighting pulsed tracer information. The presented Tool uses time as well as frequency signal processing approaches and exploits an Optical Flow analysis to extract quantitative 4D velocity vectors fields. In this work, we successfully estimate flow patterns in a nonrealistic aneurysm shaped vessel exploiting pulsed tracer information in the Flow Analysis Toolbox.

Relaxation-Based Viscosity Mapping in Different Viscous Environments

M. Utkur[*][a,b)], A. Alipour [a,b,c)], Y. Muslu [a,b)], E. U. Saritas [a,b,d)]

a) Department of Electrical and Electronics Engineering, Bilkent University, Ankara, Turkey
b) National Magnetic Resonance Research Center (UMRAM), Bilkent University, Ankara, Turkey
c) Institute of Materials Science and Nanotechnology (UNAM), Bilkent University, Ankara, Turkey
d) Neuroscience Graduate Program, Bilkent University, Ankara, Turkey
*Corresponding author, email: mustafa.utkur@bilkent.edu.tr

Magnetic Particle Imaging (MPI) has the potential to be used as a functional imaging modality. Recent color MPI studies have shown the possibility of differentiating the responses from different nanoparticles, which could be extended to differentiate nanoparticles in different environmental conditions. Our recently proposed relaxation-based viscosity mapping technique showed that relaxation time constants estimated directly from the MPI signal can provide a one-to-one mapping to viscosity. In this work, we test this viscosity mapping technique on chemically different viscous environments and compare the trends in relaxation time constants for glycerol-water mixtures and sucrose-water solutions within the biologically relevant viscosity ranges. The results show that although these two viscous environments are chemically different, the corresponding estimated time constants display identical trends, suggesting that there is a direct relation between the viscosity levels and estimated time constants, independent of the type of the medium.

Determination of the Total Circulating Blood Volume using Magnetic Particle Spectroscopy

F. Weigelt [a], A. Seifert [a], A. Kraupner [b], P. M. Jakob [a,c],
K.-H. Hiller [a,c], F. Fiedler[*] [c]

a) Department of Experimental Physics 5, University of Würzburg, Würzburg, Germany
b) nanoPET Pharma GmbH, Berlin, Germany
c) Magnetic Resonance and X-ray Imaging MRB, Development Center X-ray Technology EZRT
Fraunhofer Institute for Integrated Circuits IIS, Würzburg, Germany
*Corresponding author, email: florian.fidler@iis.fraunhofer.de

The knowledge of the patient's total blood volume is essential in clinical routine. A variety of methods have been studied over the past decades but due to its extend volume and intricate distribution throughout the body only few of them result in accurate total blood volume determination. In this work, we present a method for measuring the total blood volume based on Magnetic Particle Spectroscopy (MPS). The presented method consists of three major steps. First, from the signal-to-noise ratio (snr) estimation of the undiluted tracer and a chosen minimum accuracy of the blood volume determination combined with a rough estimation of it, a bolus volume for injection is calculated. This step has to be performed only once per used tracer. In a second step, the bolus is injected into the subject. Last, a small amount of blood is taken after a mixing time. From the measured concentration, the total blood volume is calculated with at minimum the prior given accuracy from step one.

Infinite Science
Publishing